Table of Contents

I0085856

FAT TO FABULOUS

DIET FREE WEIGHT LOSS FOR REAL WOMEN

SHARI WARE, Founder of FAB New Body

Book a complimentary 30-minute call with me to find your FABulous!
https://calendly.com/shari-ware/30min

Connect with me on Facebook: https://www.facebook.com/shariwarefab

Connect with me on my Facebook Page:
https://www.facebook.com/fabnewbody

Connect with me on Instagram:
https://www.instagram.com/shariwarefab

Connect with me on Twitter: https://twitter.com/shariwarefab

Connect with me on Linked In: https://www.linkedin.com/in/shariware

1 Best Selling Author of Healthy! Beautiful Inside & Out

You can get the book here: https://amzn.to/2V1LXfg

FEATURED IN...

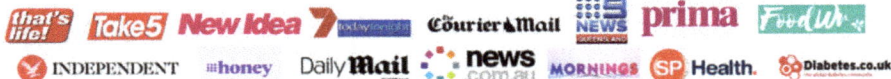

DISCLAIMER

The people and events described and depicted in this book are for educational purposes only. While every attempt has been made to verify information provided in this book, the author assumes no responsibility for any errors, inaccuracies or omissions.

If advice concerning medical matters is needed, the services of a qualified professional should be sought. This book is not intended for use as a source of medical advice.

The examples within this book are not intended to represent or guarantee that everyone or anyone will achieve their desired results. Each individual's success will be determined by his or her desire, dedication, effort and motivation. There are no guarantees you will achieve your desired outcome; the tools, stories and information are provided as examples only.

First Edition 2018 | Copyright 2018 by Shari Ware

Introduction

Do you wake up in the morning with a feeling of dread because you know when you put your feet on the floor for the first time, it's going to hurt so much you want to cry? Are you constantly held back because you're so overweight it's not physically possible to participate? Do you ever go to bed at night wondering if you'll even wake up the next day? In 2010 and for many years prior to that, that life was mine.

Maybe this is your life, too. Maybe not to the same extent, but morbidly obese is morbidly obese, no matter the actual numbers on the scale. I have written this book in the hopes of helping anyone who is in the same desperately dark place that I was and is looking for the way out. I want it to be one of those motivational books, one of those inspirational true stories that gives people that light bulb moment that enables them to change their own life.

There is definitely a way. I know because I found it. It may not be the way you thought though. It's not all about nutrition and exercise I can assure you, as you will find out when you read my story.

First of all, let's talk about the word "fat".

I don't like the word fat. It's a horrible word. So why is it included in the title of my book? I've included it because it's what I was. Let me clarify that a little more though.

There are 2 kinds of "big", which is the word I've always actually used. The first kind is the person that identifies as "big", or "big boned", or however they like to put it. They're the person who looks in the mirror and likes what they see. They're the women who are a larger size, but they have confidence, style, that little bit of sass and they strut their stuff with pride. As they should!

Then there are big people that are "fat". When they look in the mirror, they definitely do NOT like what they see. They call themselves all kinds of horrible names - fat included. They do NOT feel good. They sit on the sidelines of life. They don't let people take photos or videos of them.

I used to be FAT. Now I'm FABulous and I love every single day of the amazing life I lead.

So, if you're "fat", this book is definitely for you. By the time you've finished this book you'll be so empowered, motivated energized and inspired to find YOUR FABulous, you'll never think, imagine or feel "fat" ever again!

Some might think this book is all about me tooting my own horn. It's really not. To be quite honest, there are some things in this book that are *embarrassing* and not many people in my life actually know about. I've been brutally open and honest writing this book for one reason - I want the "fat" people reading this book to truly KNOW that I understand. I GET it! Because I've been there, too. Unless you've lived that miserable existence, you really can't appreciate how utterly debilitating it is at times.

In chapter 1, you'll learn the REAL reason why you retain weight, and I can guarantee it's not what you think it is. At the end of chapters 1 – 3, I have outlined the most important keys to successful weight release.

Chapter 2 is about showing you that YOU can change your story. It's the beginning of showing you the way and it's that first glimmer of hope. You'll also learn the first of the two most important things you MUST address if you want to successfully release your weight.

Chapter 3 is designed to fully ignite the fire of hope and belief in you. It's about some of the amazing things I have done after my 100kg weight release journey. I was offered some exciting opportunities and I set myself some massive physical challenges – just because I could! They were challenges that I never in a million years thought I would be capable of attempting or would even *want* to do.

I want you to know that absolutely anything is possible. Your current situation does NOT have to be where your story ends.

It's about inspiring you by showing you what can be achieved when you truly believe it's possible. In chapter 3, you'll learn the second of the two most important things you MUST address if you want to find YOUR FABulous!

If you want to cut to the chase and get to the chapter that's all about you, then Chapter 4 is the important one. Here you will find my step by step guide of how you can do exactly what I have done. No matter how much weight you have to release, know that this process will work no matter how many kilos you want gone forever.

My step by step guide is not going to be what you expect. As I said earlier, releasing weight is not all about nutrition and exercise. I have listed my top 31 tips in order of priority and it's a total mind, body, spirit approach. There are so many things that impact our bodies that I teach when I work with clients, but for those wanting to make a start, there is more than enough to get you moving in the right direction in this book.

One of the biggest lessons I learned on my own journey is the hardest step to take is that very first one. Once you take that step, the next one comes and the next one comes and each one gets easier and easier. If you're ready to change YOUR story for good... if you're ready to go from Fat to FABulous... then your first step is reading this book!

I absolutely know there's an amazing new life for you out there. A life that you'll LOVE!

So what are you waiting for Ms FABulous? Let's get your transformation started... see you on the inside!

Chapter One

The How and Why of It All

I used to weigh over 180kg. That's as big as a baby elephant – according to a journalist who did a story about my weight loss. My highest recorded weight was 170.2kg and I know at one point I was quite a bit heavier than that. I didn't have a set of scales at home that went higher than 150kg and I was too scared and embarrassed to go anywhere else to get weighed.

I was morbidly obese according to all the scales. I was fat. Not "phat"... "FAT"! I never used that word though. I still have trouble using that word in any context other than the fat content in food, because it was ME for so many years of my life – and I didn't like that it was me. I always used the term 'big', even now – but I was FAT, plainly and simply, FAT.

I've been big almost all my life – there's that word again! I was born on the 13th of June 1975 in Tenant Creek, Australia and I think I started to put on weight from about the age of 5. Chocolates, lollies, cakes and anything else yummy was never safe from me. My love affair with chocolate began when I was young and I don't think it will ever end.

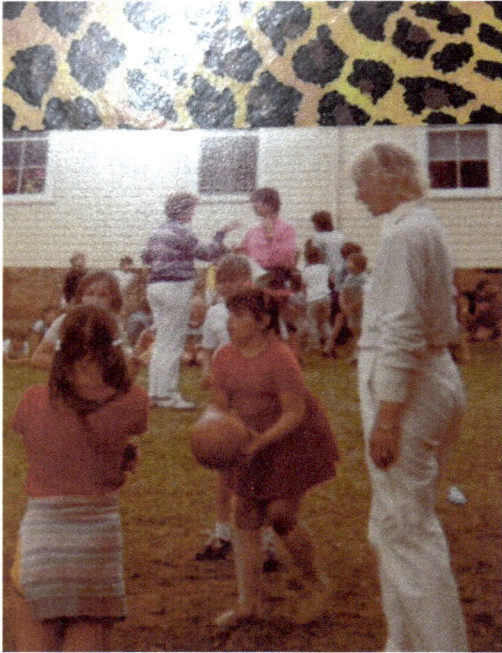

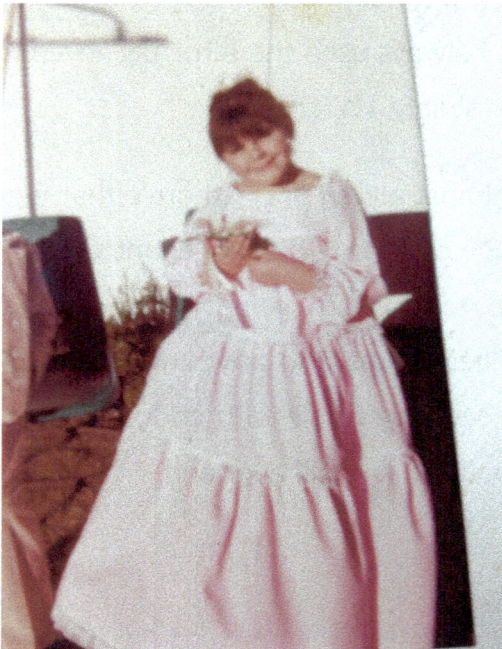

Let's start with my school years. They were horrible! My mother made my uniforms for me, and although it was to save money, it would have been hard to find them to fit me unless they were custom made anyway. I hated participating in any form or exercise, dance or sport at school because kids would stare and laugh at me, and so I found any way I could to get out of it. I was lucky that I was fairly well liked by my immediate peers and so didn't cop a lot of teasing from them, but other kids that didn't know me were not kind.

I remember one incident that was absolutely mortifying. Due to our school uniform consisting of a knee length skirt, in winter we were allowed to wear pantyhose so our legs didn't get so cold. Travelling home on the bus one day I had to stand in the aisle because all the seats were full. There were some kids from another school sitting in the seats either side of me, who spent the whole bus ride calling me names and pulling threads in my pantyhose. By the time I got off the bus I had tears streaming down my face, my pantyhose were ripped to shreds, and I had the horrible things they had said to me ringing in my ears. By the time I got home I was sobbing so hard, I couldn't speak and it took a while for my mum to calm me down and tell her what happened.

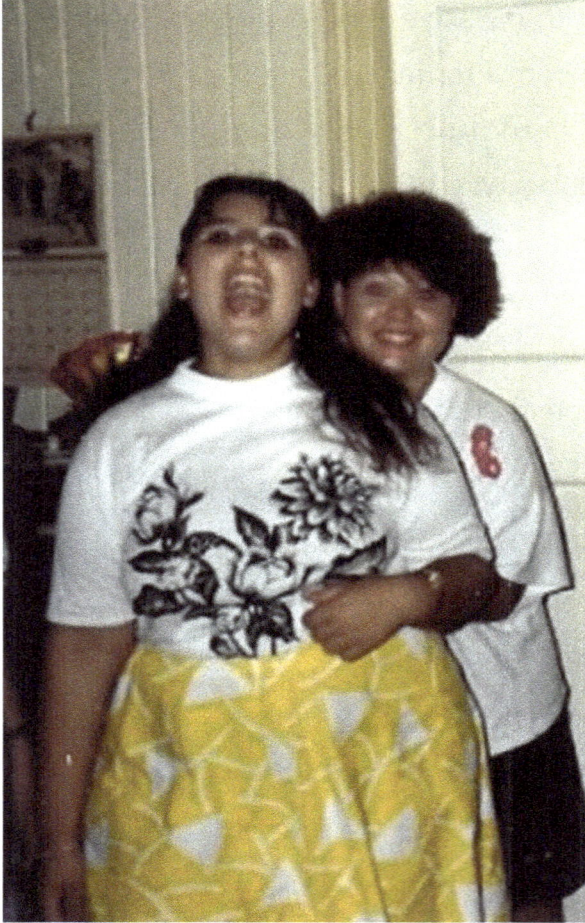

My school years – look at those clothes!

Over my school years I slowly got bigger and bigger. My parents and teachers tried all sorts of things to encourage me to lose weight, but to no avail. Even though my mum tried to limit my food intake, I would find ways to eat in secret so people didn't realise how much I was eating. We ate a lot of rice at home and I love my rice. My mum also made a lot of homemade cakes for my stepdad, and I would sneak a piece whenever there was no one around. I would cut a bit off the entire edge of the cake, so no one realized there was a piece missing.

I had such an addiction to food that I became sneaky. I'm not proud of it, but it's what I did. My mum was a shift worker, and quite often wasn't home in the afternoons after school, so it was easy for me to eat things that I shouldn't have been eating. My after school snack would be a packet of 2-minute noodles with butter and cheese melted through it. We had pasta a lot as well, which is another thing I love and tended to eat too much of. Being so inactive of course only exacerbated the problem.

When I was half way through year 11, I went on a 12-month student exchange to the States. I lived with a host family and attended Senior Year in the local high school. Although this was a wonderful experience, I was introduced to a range of junk food I'd never dreamed possible and of course I wanted to try all of it. That year didn't do any good for my weight problem and contributed to me tipping the scales at around 100kg by the time I graduated grade 12 in Australia at the end of 1992. It was only the fact that I was an Aussie and a novelty for people that saved me from being bullied at my school in the US.

I had never been asked out by anyone my age because of my weight. I had always been told that I had the prettiest face. You know the phrase, "Such a pretty face - shame about the body". Nobody ever said the second part of that phrase to me directly, but I always knew they thought it and I added it on in my head every. single. time.

I guess it was due to my low self esteem that I could never see beauty when I looked in the mirror. Occasionally I would catch a glimpse of it, but what I saw in the mirror most of the time was definitely not my version of pretty. It was horrible, it was ugly – *I* was ugly.

After I turned 18, I decided I really wanted a boyfriend and so endeavoured to try to lose some weight. I joined a gym, exercised almost every day and watched what I ate. I started to lose weight and became addicted to seeing those results, starving myself to get even better results. I remember at one point I was only eating one meal every second day and the rest of the time I just drank water.

I lost around 40kg and got down to a size 12, but I was lucky I didn't do major damage to my health. I was young and uneducated about how the body works, and will never ever do that to my body again. Carrying too much weight is certainly unhealthy, but so is starving your body of the nutrients it needs to survive. Both are at the wrong ends of the spectrum and both will cause health problems eventually. It's only a matter of time.

I had a bit of fun for a while with my girlfriends. We would go out to the nightclubs every week and party. However, while losing the weight and finally becoming attractive to the opposite sex boosted my self esteem, I still lacked a lot of confidence and it didn't take much to knock down the little that I had.

I had a couple of short term boyfriends and then I met my partner. Eventually we did what most young couples do and moved in together and everything was wonderful. After about 12 months I became pregnant with our daughter and began to put on weight with the pregnancy, which was the beginning of our problems.

Everybody assured me I would release the weight after she was born, but I struggled. I hadn't learned to release the weight the right way the first time around, and so I found it hard to release it after the birth. Once again I saw an ugly person in the mirror. I felt so unattractive that I continually questioned in my mind whether my partner still loved me. I didn't love myself, so how could he? It wasn't something I could hide forever and I told him my fears, which of course he assured me were silly.

One thing I can honestly say is that even when I was at 140kg toward the end of our relationship, my partner never once put me down or said anything negative to me about my weight. The only bad thing he ever said to me about it once, when he was very angry and frustrated with me, was that if I was so unhappy about it, then either do something about it or get over it. Which isn't bad at all – he was really just saying it like it was, and he was right.

What people don't realise is, we don't believe it's as easy as that. Add in the pressures of being young parents (I just turned 20 and my partner was almost 20 when we had our daughter), a young baby, financial pressures, lack of social life due to a young baby, and it's not hard to figure out why we didn't last. By far the biggest issue though was my weight because of how it made me feel about myself and how I imagined that made my partner feel about me.

My partner and I were together for a total of 9 years and although we had many happy times, we also had quite a few struggles. As a result my weight was like a yoyo. I would lose some weight, and then something would happen and I would go off the rails and put back on what I'd lost and more. Over time I once again got bigger and bigger, and by the time we separated permanently I was around 140kg. Over the next eight or so years, I continued to yoyo and grew heavier and heavier, until I hit that final tipping point and was able to turn my life around.

When my partner and I separated for the final time (we had separated quite a few times over the years), I decided I needed to make a clean break and moved with my daughter from Cairns to Brisbane. I found a job on the Gold Coast and after I had been working there for a while I decided to become a foster carer. It was something I'd always wanted to do but didn't know you could be a single parent foster carer. I was a foster carer for 7 years and had mostly teenage girls that could fit into our lifestyle and be a companion for my daughter.

I remember how so many simple things were just so hard for me when I was at my biggest. Things that normal people wouldn't even realize could ever be a problem. Like having to get down on my hands and knees if I dropped a pen. For most people it would be a two second exercise. For me it would take at least a couple of minutes and would involve a lot of pain and effort. By the time I was sitting back on my chair anyone walking into my office would have thought I'd just done a 100 metre sprint! I can laugh about it now – but it's an embarrassed laugh, not a happy one.

I had to either walk sideways down the hallway at work or duck into a doorway when I saw someone coming the other way because I was so big I was almost the width of the hallway. I felt like I needed one of those wide load signs! I had to do that for so many years that sometimes I still do it now out of habit and people remind me that I don't have to do that anymore.

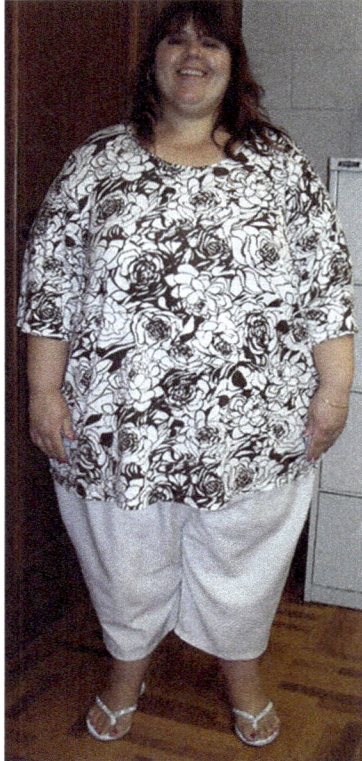

My first progress photo!

I hated going anywhere, especially places where there were lots of people. I always felt like I was being watched – like I was such a freak that people couldn't help but stare at me with a varying range of expressions – horror, disgust, pity, disdain. I always felt as if I was being judged and found extremely lacking. I felt sorry for my children and I actually remember one instance where I apologised to my daughter for any embarrassment that I may have ever caused her. I was absolutely serious. I felt like a total embarrassment to not only myself, but most of all to my family. They loved me unconditionally of course, but that's the way I felt at the time.

One year when my partner and I were together, we went on a holiday with our daughter and we went on a 3D ride at a theme park. One of those where you sit on a chair and the movie on the screen is so real it's like you're a part of it. It was a simulated ride as well so there were bars that came down and locked in place in front of you, just like a roller coaster. I didn't know about the bar until after we had sat down and so when the bar started lowering, I kept praying it would be ok.

Of course it wasn't. I was so big the bar couldn't lock in place, even though they tried a few times. Of course while they were trying, everyone was watching and finally they asked me if I could move to a chair at the back of the room that didn't have a bar. I had to leave my partner and daughter where they were and walk to the back of the room with everyone watching me – judging me, feeling sorry for me, disgusted in me – that's what I felt they were thinking because that's what I thought about myself. I've had many embarrassing moments in my life as a result of my weight, but that's one that really stands out as one of the worst.

I hated to travel. Most people love to travel. I hated it and dreaded every time I had to fly somewhere. I would always make sure I could take my daughter with me and I would book us seats together, with her in the middle seat and myself in the window seat. That way, we could put the arm rest between us in the up position, as I was so big it was very uncomfortable to have it down.

After we got into our seats, my daughter would always go up to a flight attendant and very quietly ask for a seat belt extender for me. The seat belt would not even go near me and I was too embarrassed to ask for one myself. Going to the toilet was also a no go – there was no way I was going to fit in that tiny cubicle. I always made sure I went to the toilet just before I got on the flight and didn't leave my seat until it was time to disembark. I also waited for everyone else to get off before I did, so people didn't watch me have to walk sideways down the aisle because I was too big to fit front on.

I could rarely find any clothes off the rack that fit or looked any good on me. I'm extremely lucky that my mother is a dressmaker and made most of my clothes for me. I have no idea what size I ended up because of that, but it was definitely enormous by anyone's standards.

One of my worst memories was when I was moving cities and I knew I would need some professional looking clothes for job interviews. My mum didn't have time to make them for me and so she told me she was taking me shopping. I begged and pleaded with her because I knew it was going to be a horrible experience, but she insisted it would be fine and dragged me to the shops with my sister.

We did find some things that looked presentable, but it took a lot of trying on. I remember at one point standing in the changing room sobbing uncontrollably because I had tried on so many things that were either too small or just looked downright disgusting on me because I was trying to squash an elephant into a potato sack!

It's embarrassing to admit, but even the simple act of going to the toilet was a task at times. I was so big that it was hard to wipe my backside. I even had trouble fitting into toilets that were smaller than the norm. That was another reason I didn't like to go anywhere. I had my comfort zones where I knew I wouldn't have an issue and I stuck to them as much as I could.

Even the very first thing that every single person does every single day when they get out of bed was so very, very hard for me. I got so big, that when I rolled myself out of bed in the morning - I did literally have to roll because I was so massive - and put my feet on the floor, I had to brace myself for the pain that was coming. I had to sit on the side of my bed, wiggle down to the end (as much as an elephant can wiggle), grit my teeth and pull myself up via the corner post of my bed.

Every single day it was the same. When my feet took the weight of my body for the first time in the morning, I couldn't help but cry because it hurt so much. I couldn't move until my feet adjusted to the massive weight I had just placed on them. It would take a good couple of minutes for the pain to subside. It was one of the things I dreaded most every day - the simple act of putting my feet on the floor first thing in the morning. How sad is that?!

So how and why did I get to that point? It took me a long time to realise that I was an emotional eater. When I'm upset, angry, stressed, depressed –it makes me want to eat and drink. It's a vicious cycle that's extremely hard to break and one that took me about 20 years to finally learn how to deal with. While I still have the urge at times to emotionally eat, I've learned to control myself a whole lot better. I still have times where I make a conscious choice to indulge the emotional eater within myself, but I'm always aware of it now and it's definitely a choice that I make consciously.

There are a few things that have contributed to my emotional eating over the years. My mother has battled a weight problem for most of her life, as has my father. Unfortunately for me, it runs in both sides of my family.

Over the last few years I have learned a lot. One of the things I've learned is scientifically, there are 3 different body types and what you eat and how you exercise can be much more effective depending on the body type you have. It didn't surprise me at all that I had what I consider to be the most challenging one and it actually explained a lot about why my body reacts the way it does to certain foods and of course, they're the foods I love the most. So when we combine these factors with a love of chocolate, lollies, cakes, rice, pasta, potatoes – pretty much anything that's bad for you when eaten in large quantities – there we have one of the biggest reasons why I began to put on weight over the years.

I also had several instances of being sexually abused as a child. I don't feel it necessary to be too detailed about those instances, but I am mentioning them because they led to me experiencing feelings of shame, guilt, unworthiness and undeserving of anything good in my life. Those feelings and beliefs led to emotional eating and I carried them through most of my life.

As I grew bigger and bigger, I was teased and called names. People were constantly telling me I shouldn't eat this and I shouldn't eat that and I needed to lose weight, and even though it was because they cared about me, it still made me feel horrible. This caused me to eat more, because in the short term, it made me feel better – and so the vicious cycle began. I would be angry, hurt, upset or depressed because of my weight and how that impacted on the rest of my life, so I would eat, which would make me fatter and the situation worse.

What also became more and more damaged over time was my self esteem. Not only were other people calling me names and putting me down, I did it to myself. By the time I was 18, I had very little self esteem. People observing me would never have guessed, because the person I presented to the world was happy and smiling. So many overweight people are happy and smiling. It's a bit of a stereotype really. The happy and smiling picture that I presented to the world hid a very sad person inside. A person that hated themselves and the fact they were so weak they couldn't control what they put in their mouth and couldn't get off their backside to do some exercise.

It took me a long time to understand the reason why no matter how much I tried to change my habits, I just couldn't stick to it. I remember watching one of the first series of the Australian version of The Biggest Loser. I'd never watched the US version. I actually didn't even know it was a weight loss show. I thought it was just about people that were really big losers in the US, and since I knew what it felt like to be the brunt of people's jokes, that kind of show certainly wasn't going to be on my watch list!

Once I realized what it was and that there was an Australian series coming out I was excited to watch it. I thought maybe it could help me to release weight somehow. I loved the show and watched every episode religiously. In one episode I remember Jillian was having a heart to heart with one of the contestants trying to get to the reason why they were big. He kept telling her he didn't know, and she told him he did. Somewhere deep down inside, there was a psychological reason why people who didn't have a medical issue that made them retain weight, had a weight problem. The contestant didn't have a medical problem, so she insisted it had to be psychological. Together they talked it out and although I can't remember what his reason was, he eventually realized what it was and was able to move forward on his journey much better.

What Jillian said made sense to me. Apparently I didn't have a medical problem other than some challenging genes, so maybe my problem was psychological...

The problem with psychological issues is that even though we know we have one, we don't always know what it is. Sometimes we do things that we don't understand. We wonder to ourselves, "Why did I do that?" or "What am I doing?" A lot of times it seems inconsequential and so we don't delve further into it and quickly forget about it.

Weighing in at 180kg meant that as much as I wanted to bury my head in the sand, I really needed to try and figure out what was going on in my head. So I started to analyse my life on a day to day basis. I didn't sit and think for hours on end – I didn't have time. I was and still am a very busy person. There is ALWAYS something for me to be doing. Even at the size of a baby elephant, one of my family described me back then (and still does today), as the busiest person she knows. I just continued to go about my daily life with the psychological thing in the back of my mind and thought about it whenever I had the chance.

The conclusion I came to after about six months sounded absolutely ridiculous even to me. It seemed so ridiculous that I promptly discounted it and kept looking for other reasons. Over a period of another couple of months though, I kept coming back to the same conclusion and it started to make more sense to me – and in the end I proved myself right. I finally came to the realization that the reason I wasn't being successful at releasing weight was because......are you ready for it?.....drum roll please......

I didn't want another relationship!

I know, I know! Utterly ridiculous! As I said, I thought so too at first. Yet every time I thought about it, it made more and more sense. I can hear you asking how on earth not wanting another relationship could possibly keep someone from releasing weight? As ridiculous as it sounds, it's extremely possible. The unconscious mind does exactly what we tell it to do, whether we're telling it consciously or unconsciously.

You see, when I was younger I was a big girl and unattractive to those of the opposite sex. Then I lost the weight and that all changed. So in my subconscious mind, if I made myself as unattractive to the opposite sex as I could, then I wouldn't have to deal with any attention that I wasn't ready for. It was my personal protective suit of armour, designed to protect my very vulnerable heart. It worked extremely well for a long time.

But why? Why not just fend off any unwanted attention? That would be the right way to deal with the issue. That would be *logical*. Unfortunately, it wasn't a conscious thing and it took me a long time to realise that's what I was doing. Even once I did realise it, I found it hard to do something about my weight because I still didn't want a relationship and so I would sabotage myself without realizing it until it was too late.

My armour of fat helped me to hide from the world. It helped me to withdraw from social situations. I didn't get asked to a lot of social occasions because most people knew that although I would say yes out of politeness, I didn't really want to attend. It was another of those vicious cycles. I didn't want to be a part of the world because I didn't want to take the chance of going through the pain of a relationship again and so my fat suit helped me to hide. However, not being a part of the world made me unhappy and so I would emotionally eat. To the world I projected a façade of happiness, which was definitely not how I was feeling inside.

SHARI'S FAB SECRET KEY TO SUCCESS

If you're overweight, it's because of things buried deep in your subconscious. The key to long-term weight release is to work on what's going on in your head. When you get your head in the right space, you CAN achieve anything!

"To shift your life in a desired direction, you must powerfully shift your subconscious." ~ Kevin Michel

Chapter Two

Change is A Beautiful Thing

So what changed? A lot! There are a few big reasons why I was finally able to turn my life around, but by far the biggest one proved beyond all doubt that I was right about the reason for my weight problem in the first place. It's an important reason, but it definitely should not have been the *most* important. My other reasons were far more important, but the mind is very powerful and although they should have been enough, they weren't.

My daughter was a couple of years away from turning 18 and she would be spending at least a year in the US with family after she graduated. I suddenly realised one day she was going to be off overseas on her exciting adventure, which I was ecstatic about for her, but I was going to be alone, on the couch, with no life.

I'd spent my years hiding from the world doing everything I could for my children, family and friends. My children all attended dancing, cheerleading, karate and different school events. Our days were always busy trying to fit everything in and I spent a lot of time in the car driving them from one thing to the other in between work and whatever else had to be done. I knew I didn't want to be a foster carer forever. I had no set timeframe at that point, but I did know that one day I would be done. And then I would be alone, on the couch, with no life.

I didn't want to be alone and I didn't want to be raising children my whole life. I realised that I was finally ready to put myself out there romantically again, and I wasn't getting any younger. I was 34 years old and I had at least 100kg to release, maybe more. That wasn't going to happen overnight. It was going to take me at least a couple of years doing it the right way, maybe more.

By the time I released the weight I would be at least 36, if not older. I also knew that up until that point I had been extremely lucky with my health. Doctors were always amazed when they took my blood pressure and told me that for such an obese person, my blood pressure was excellent. Thank goodness for THOSE genes!

Despite the fact that I had been lucky up to that point, I knew that one day my luck was bound to run out. You can't put that amount of strain on your body and expect it to go on forever. My daughter being so close to 18 made me start thinking about the fact that she was not only going to be leaving me, but she would be going through all the experiences of life; meeting someone, falling in love, getting married, having children. I wanted to see all of that. I wanted to be a part of it. Which was *not* going to happen if I died from a heart attack, which was where I was headed. I had absolutely no doubt about that. It was only a matter of time. I was literally a walking, talking heart attack. A ticking time bomb which could go off at any time and I am so very lucky to be here today.

At first it was a slow process. A very slow process! At the beginning of 2010 I made a silent promise to myself that it would be the year I started to release my weight forever. I rejoined a weight release group that I had been a member of in the past and tried to follow their plan again. Their weight release plan was very good; the food variety was excellent and the basic concept promotes eating mostly fresh fruits and vegetables, whole grains, dairy and lean meats, with allowances for occasional treats. They had a system to keep track of how much you could eat each day to make sure you had a weight release each week, which was usually the result if you stuck to the plan.

My problem was I could lie to myself very easily when it came to portion size. Maybe *lie* is a bit harsh. Maybe denial is a better way to describe it. I could be *in denial* when it came to portion size. I could serve up what I thought was a serving of rice, but if I actually measured it, it would more likely be at least 2, if not 3 servings. I did this with a lot of food. I just love food. I love the taste of it and I love the way it makes me feel when I eat it. A lot of people don't realise that food can be an addiction and with me it definitely was. Food can be as addictive to some people as drugs, alcohol or cigarettes. Which makes it harder to learn to control it.

Think about it - you can live without drugs, alcohol or cigarettes. You can beat the addiction and then only have to keep yourself away from it. It's not easy I know, but it's easier than trying to control a food addiction. You can't keep yourself away from food. You *have* to eat food to live. If you give up food entirely, you die. There's no way to get away from it. It's everywhere. It's part of our everyday life.

For that whole year I tried to follow the eating plan. I also signed up at a local Curves gym and made a concerted effort to exercise there at least 3 times per week. I got to the end of the year and had lost 10kg. I was frustrated! I had been working so hard and it took me a whole year to lose 10kg.

I got through Christmas and New Year, and on New Year's Day I sat down and decided to actually write down my goals for the year. I thought that maybe if I actually wrote them out on a piece of paper and put them somewhere where I could see them every day it would help. I didn't think it could make anything worse, that's for sure!

I had a list of 10 things and the first thing on the list was to release weight, but I made it more specific than that. I remembered the concept of SMART goals, and so I tried to do that with all of my goals. I sat and thought about the 10kg I had lost the previous year. I didn't beat myself up about it. I told myself it was a good start. It may have taken me a whole year, but I was still 10kg lighter than I had been a year before. I also told myself that at that rate, it was going to take me at least 10 years to release the weight that I needed to release and I was already 34. I had already wasted so many years of my life, I knew I needed to do better this year.

I was just over 160kg at the beginning of 2011. I decided that I really wanted to see a figure under 100kg on those scales by New Year's Eve 2011. That meant I had to release just over 60kg, as 99.9 is a number I would definitely be ecstatic about seeing. I knew it was a big goal, but I also knew that if I really wanted to, I would find a way to do it – and I really, really wanted to!

So now my goal was written down and it was time to work out a plan of action of how I was going to achieve it. I knew that while what I had been doing had been working, it was way too slow a process, and that if I was going to achieve my goal, I had to change what I was doing in a much bigger way.

I saw an ad for the Biggest Loser Club online and decided I would check it out. The Biggest Loser Club had various programs that you could follow, and after a lot of thought, I decided I would try their express program for 1 week. It meant I was limited to 1200 calories per day, but it was something I had never tried before and I figured I could do anything for 1 week. If it didn't work, I would try something else.

I have to say that I completely underestimated how hard it was going to be and I am massively understating the situation when I say that week was *hard* for me. It became clear very early on that I obviously consumed a lot more than 1200 calories on a daily basis. I had certain guidelines I had to follow in conjunction with the 1200 calorie limit to ensure my nutrition was optimized. I had to have a certain amount of protein, carbs and fat per day, which left very little scope for anything other than healthy food that would help me to reach those targets.

I have to say that week was not the most pleasant for my children or workmates either. I was having massive withdrawals from food, I was tired and I was HANGRY!! My body was receiving more than enough food, but my mind and body still craved a lot more than I was feeding it. If I didn't know it before that week, by the end of it there was absolutely no doubt in my mind that food was definitely an addiction for me.

Towards the end of the week I was torn between the two possible outcomes. On the one hand I hoped I had a good result on the scales because I really wanted all the sacrifices I had made to be worth it. But on the other hand I hoped it didn't work because then I wouldn't have to continue with it and could try something else that wasn't as hard.

Weigh in day came and I finally stood on the scales to find that I had released a massive 5kgs. That's the most weight I had ever released before and if you averaged out my kilos released the previous year, the 5kg before that had taken me 6 months! I was so happy I cried. I had finally found something that worked for me. A system. A formula. A step by step process, which if I followed religiously should guarantee results.

I knew it was going to be hard, but I also knew that it should work, and because I knew that, it made it easier for me to do it. I would like to add here something that's very important and that I feel very passionate about. Although I released the bulk of my weight from sticking to a 1200 calorie intake on a daily basis, it is *not* what I now recommend to my clients. When I started my journey, I knew very little about nutrition and I did what worked for me at the time. I have learned a lot about nutrition over the past few years and there are much better ways of eating that provide the same results and are much healthier for our bodies. Which is what I now recommend to those I work with.

The next 12 months were some of the hardest I have ever lived through, but they were also a time of massive personal learning and growth. A time of empowerment, a time of getting to know and love myself, a time of terror and excitement and sometimes both of those at the same time.

I wanted to see that number on the scale drop again, so week after week I stuck to my 1200 calories per day. I did know though, that if I was too strict about it I wouldn't be able to keep it up, so I put some things in place so I didn't feel like I could never have any treats.

First of all, when they were on special, I would buy some of the multipacks of mini chocolate bars. Things like Snickers, Cherry Ripes, Bountys, Freddos, etc. I would keep some in the fridge and maybe two or three times a week I would let myself have one after dinner. Everyone has something food wise they don't want to give up. I can give up a lot of things, but if I ever had to give up chocolate I would be very sad. Chocolate is my thing. I don't have to have a lot of it. Even just a little bit every now and then is enough to keep me from feeling deprived, and one of those mini bars a few times a week was enough to keep me sane.

The other thing I did was schedule in a day off. In the beginning, I would schedule 1 day off every 6 weeks. Keep in mind that I was counting my calories to make sure I stuck to my 1200 calorie limit. That meant that I had to weigh, measure and record everything, and I do mean EVERYTHING that went into my mouth. It required a lot of time, effort and dedication and that was just the food portion of what I was doing to release the weight. I had a lot of help from my children, which made it a lot easier and I greatly appreciated that, but it was still a major chore. So my day off every six weeks was a day we all looked forward to.

On that day, I didn't count anything. I also allowed myself to have anything I wanted guilt free. I made sure on my day off I had things that I wouldn't normally allow myself. That didn't mean it was necessarily unhealthy. Quite often on my day off I would make sure I had pasta or rice, because I couldn't afford to eat them on a 1200 calorie day.

Once I felt I had the food under control, I started to increase my exercise. I was a member of Curves, so I made sure I did my 3 recommended sessions per week there. I also had a work colleague who saw a great offer for personal training where you paid a fixed price for the session no matter how many people attended, and asked me if I wanted to go with her and split the cost. I had wanted to try a personal trainer but I didn't feel I could afford it. This was a way that made the cost for a single parent much more affordable and I wanted to give myself every bit of support I could.

I hate wasting money and I knew that if I paid for it, I would go no matter how much I didn't want to. I also figured that going with my workmate would keep me from giving up on it as well. It worked and is one of the best things I ever did. I have come so far from when I first started exercising regularly to now, that sometimes it seems hard for me to believe it myself!

Over the course of the year I became smaller, fitter and stronger and as I progressed I started to increase my exercise. I was doing the 3 times per week at Curves, 30 minutes of Personal Training 1 day per week (which by the way felt like the longgggest 30 minutes of my entire life every single session), and then I started to add in walking which eventually turned into running.

When I first started running, I was still over 100kg. I still felt massive and hated people watching me exercise. I didn't feel attractive at the best of times and I felt even less attractive (if that was even possible) when I was exercising. I also still felt as if people were always looking at me and judging me or making fun of me.

I used to walk around a lake near where my children attended dancing classes which was almost 4km around. On the one side it was all open, but on the other side there were a few clumps of tall reeds about 10m long growing at intervals along the side of the lake. I knew that when I was walking beside the reeds, as long as there was no one behind or in front of me, no one could see me. Well that's what I thought anyway!

What I would do was walk as fast as I could around the lake and then when I was approaching a clump of reeds, I would look ahead and behind me to make sure no one was there and then run from the beginning of the reeds to just before the end and then drop back down to a walk. It's now a funny story I tell people, and it makes me laugh at myself whenever I think about it.

I didn't tell many people what I was doing in the beginning. I had tried to do this thing so many times in the past and had told people, and then when I wasn't successful it made it even worse because they all knew I was a failure just as much as I did. So I was reluctant to tell people this time around. I did go to weight release group meetings with another one of my work colleagues though, so she knew what I was doing, but I asked her to keep it a secret.

When I hit my first 10kg lost, she made me let her take a photo of me. I hated photos. I looked horrible in them and I avoided them at all costs. The truth really hurts when it's staring you in the face, and a camera tells no lies. I remember my daughter writing me a letter when she was about 10 years old, begging me to let people take photos of me. One day she knew I wouldn't be here anymore and she wanted to have as many photos of me as she could so she would have them when I was gone.

Mummy

To my dear and wonderful mother,

I'm writing this for you to tell you how much I appreciate you and how much you mean to me.

I love you so much and I know I have my moments and at times I may not seem like the perfect child At times I may not like your rules and decisions but I know that they are there for a reason and I abide by because I love you too much to disobey you.

You mean so much to me that if something were to happen to you I don't know what I would do. You are so good to me even though I may not deserve it at times and I cherish every moment I have with you. I know you hate cameras but I need photos of you because one day you're not going to be there for me and then what am I going to have to remember my wonderful, loving and beautiful mummy by.

Thank you for everything that you do for me and everything you give to me even though it may seem that I don't appreciate it just know that deep down inside I really do appreciate it!

Love always...
Your only loving, understanding and beautiful daughter Nataasjia Marina Leilani Williams

I was so heartbroken when I read that letter from my daughter. Of course she was right, but even with that playing on my mind every time someone wanted to take a photo, I still struggled to allow it. I finally gave in to my workmate though and she took my first photo when I was about 160kg. When I had lost another 10kg, she made me let her take another one. I was still reluctant, but not quite as reluctant as I had been previously. People were starting to notice by this stage and started to ask me if I had released weight. If I was asked the question directly, I would answer in the affirmative, but I was still reluctant to volunteer the information.

By the time I had released 30kgs, there was no reluctance about having a photo taken or telling people. I had finally proved to myself that I was really doing this thing and raced in to work to have my photo taken with such excitement, literally bursting at the seams to tell everyone I had made another milestone! My workmate continued to take a photo every 10kg lost and at certain important milestones along the way, and I am so grateful to her for making me do that. It still amazes me when I see all those photos lined up from start to finish. The smile became wider and wider with each and every one. It really was like the transformation of a caterpillar to a beautiful butterfly. Even more amazing was the fact that I was actually starting to feel beautiful, too!

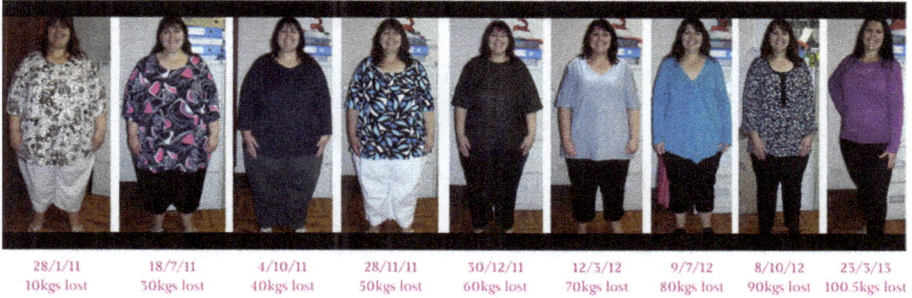

| 28/1/11 | 18/7/11 | 4/10/11 | 28/11/11 | 30/12/11 | 12/3/12 | 9/7/12 | 8/10/12 | 23/3/13 |
| 10kgs lost | 30kgs lost | 40kgs lost | 50kgs lost | 60kgs lost | 70kgs lost | 80kgs lost | 90kgs lost | 100.5kgs lost |

As I released more and more weight, a whole new world began to appear to me. Every so often I would hit a new milestone. Simple things such as not having intense pain shoot through my feet the first time I put them on the floor in the morning. Being able to sit in a chair with arms comfortably. No longer having to be picky about where I went to the toilet because I could fit better. Being able to buy proper shoes and not have to wear thongs all the time because that's pretty much all I could afford that would fit my fat feet. Being able to get down on my knees on the floor and up again without it taking a lot of time, effort and energy. Not having to ask for a seat belt extender on an airplane. These are things that most people take for granted because they've never been massively obese and had the problems associated with it. It's not a pleasant experience and I was so ecstatically happy that I was finally succeeding at changing my life.

My goal for 2011 was to release 60kg. It was a massive goal and not surprisingly, I didn't make it. At my final weigh in for the year on 30/11/2011, I hit another milestone and made it to 60kg released, which meant I had lost 50kg for the year. I aimed for the stars and I didn't quite make it, but I got a lot further than if I hadn't aimed for them in the first place! The sense of pride and achievement I had in myself was indescribable and I celebrated the New Year with excited anticipation for what it would hold for me.

On New Year's Day 2012, I looked back and reflected on the year gone by with all of its ups and downs, blood, sweat and tears, milestones and triumphs. I now had a new appreciation of just what I could achieve if I really put my mind to it. Once again, I took the time to sit down and write out my goals and really cement them in my mind. I had come a long way but I was far from finished!

The first week of 2012 I took as a rest week. I had been working hard for a really long time and I had at least another year of hard work to go, so I had planned to have the first week of the new year off. I didn't go crazy, but I didn't weigh and measure my food, I wasn't as strict with it and I didn't exercise. It did me the world of good. But it definitely had a negative impact on my body. I had thought that it would, but I needed that reminder. It was a valuable exercise for me because it refreshed in my mind just how quickly I could put the weight back on if I went back to my old ways.

Week two of 2012 I was raring to go again and set about getting back into my routine of good nutrition and exercise. The first couple of days back at Curves were a bit tough after a week of no activity and pretty crappy eating, but I soon started to feel better. Not too far into the year, another colleague of mine asked me about group sessions that were run at the Fitness Enhancement where I did my personal training and it got me thinking.

I was able to do a lot more by that stage compared to when I first started my personal training and my contracted sessions were almost finished. I enquired about the group sessions and discovered I could go to as many as I liked during the week for the same price as it cost me to do one 30 minute private session per week. The group sessions were 45 minutes long and they had several over the course of every day so plenty to choose from. There was no reason why I couldn't get to at least a couple each week if not more. So once my contracted PT sessions finished, I "graduated" to their group sessions and haven't looked back since.

On the 3rd of August 2012 I hit my next major milestone. I weighed in at 85.1kg, meaning I had lost exactly half of my body weight. I couldn't have planned it better if I tried! The lady didn't know why I was so excited when I hopped on the scale. I knew it would be close. I had been trying for a while to get to that next magic number. I could hardly contain myself while she recorded the number and as soon as she had I hopped off the scale and was jumping up and down with joy and tears welling in my eyes.

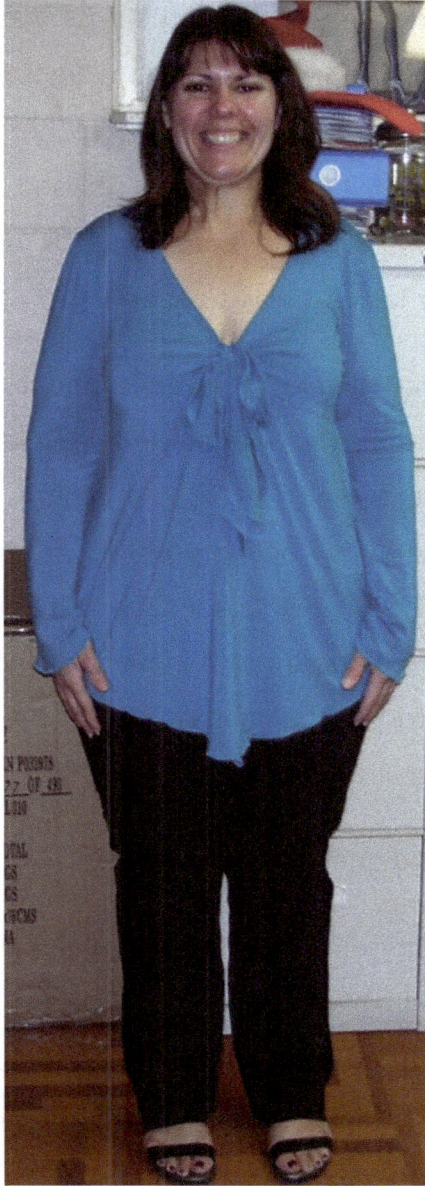

Half my body weight released!

Another lady asked me what all the fuss was about and all I could do was point out my current weight and total weight released figures in my record book. It took her a few minutes to comprehend it, but when she finally realised what I had done she gave me a big hug and excitedly took my book to show some of the other ladies. I was so happy!

It was around that time I received a phone call from a lady named Roula Pontifix who was the Public Relations Manager of SP Health Co who owned The Biggest Loser Club Online. Roula said she could see by my online profile that I had released a lot of weight using The Biggest Loser Club and wanted to know if I would be willing to be participate in a photo shoot and interview process for my story to be used as one of their success stories and for promotions.

Ummmmm... stupid question... hell yeah!

I tried to contain myself as much as I could while I was talking to her, but after I hung up the phone I started jumping up and down in excitement. The photo shoot wasn't going to be until after the new year, but it gave me something awesome to look forward to and work towards. I still had weight to release and I wanted to be a lot smaller before I got to that photo shoot!

October 6th 2012 saw me reach another milestone with total kilos released to date of 92.1kg. Reaching the 90kg released mark started me thinking about the next milestone which was going to be massive. 100kg. My weight release had been slowing. It was getting harder. I was getting tired. I had also discovered "fun" and that meant that I had a lot more temptation around me that I gave into at times, making my weight release more difficult and much slower.

There were only a few months left of the year and I really wanted to reach that extra special magic number by New Year's Eve of 2012. October 13th, 93.7kg released. October 27th, 95.2kg released. November 15th, 98.7kg released. For the rest of November and all of December 2012 I tried so very, very hard to get to that magic number. I wanted it so badly and it was so close, but always just out of reach.

Once again I didn't make my goal for the year. I was disappointed but I refused to go to an official weigh in until I was positive that I would see that magical number on the scale under my feet. New Year's Eve came and I celebrated as I had the previous year and made a vow to myself that whatever it took, I would see that magic number not too far into the New Year. I knew I would make that next extra magical milestone. It might take me a bit longer, but I was determined to get there!

New Year had now become a ritual for me, and it will forever be a ritual that I will keep because it was the beginning of the monumentous change I made in my life. On New Year 's Day I once again took the day to reflect upon the year that was past and set my goals for the one just beginning. Number one on the list was that magic number of 100kg released. I had a photo shoot coming up and I wanted to be looking as good as I could. I only had 1.3kg to go to get to that magic number, but sometimes when you're trying really hard to achieve something, it seems to be just out of reach.

The photo shoot was planned for the end of March and it came right down to the wire. On the 23rd March 2013 I weighed in at 69.7kg and couldn't speak for the tears of joy streaming down my face. I made two milestones that day. Not only did I make it to 100.5kg released, but I made it to the 60's. I was under 70kg. Oh what a feeling! Words cannot ever describe how I felt that day and it brings tears to my eyes every single time I remember it!

Who would ever have imagined that I could ever get as far as I had, let alone achieve such a wondrously magic milestone. I was so proud of the fact that I had managed to come so far. That I had managed to pull myself out of the dark abyss of pain and despair that was my life previously. I am so joyously happy that I was able to do that and I hate to think what would have happened if I hadn't.

SHARI'S FAB SECRET KEY TO SUCCESS

Finding your "Why Power" is vital for successful long term weight release. Not only is it important to have strong "whys", but also to identify and counteract your "why nots". If your "why nots" outweigh your "whys", it will be much more difficult to release the weight.

"You can't fix a why to problem with a how to answer."
~ Noah St John

Chapter Three

An Amazing New Life

The 12 months following my last epic weigh in were a whirlwind of amazing experiences which began with my photoshoot with The Biggest Loser Club Australia. I was flown to Sydney in the morning and caught a taxi to the location. I got to meet some other lovely ladies who had also lost varying amounts of weight using The Biggest Loser Club. I got to try on and was photographed in some lovely clothes and styled by a stylist. I was treated to the whole hair and makeup experience and could hardly hold back the tears as I looked in the mirror and saw a beautiful face staring back at me. I didn't even recognize myself. I had to remind myself that was my own face staring back at me. That beautiful face that didn't look like mine.

Posing in heels is hard! I kept feeling like I was going to topple over if I breathed too hard during a pose. Turn your head slightly up and right, stay there but put your left hand on your hip... slide it round to the back a bit further... now turn your right toe to the left slightly... If I ever thought a model had an easy job, I certainly have a new found respect for them. I enjoyed every minute of it though. I could definitely do more of that I reckon!

The day seemed to go by so fast. Photo after photo was taken, we had a lovely lunch in between and before I knew it, it was time to go back to the airport and I was on a flight back home. I will always remember it as one of the most exciting days of my life and the beginning of many more exciting experiences that came about through my affiliation with The Biggest Loser Club Australia.

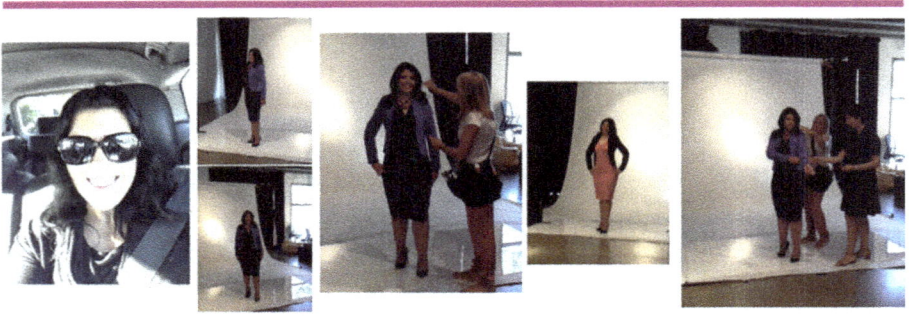

Roula contacted me a little while after the photoshoot to say that Today Tonight wanted to do a story on me. They came to my house on the 12th April 2013 to film the story. Once again I had to have my hair and makeup done. I could definitely get used to that! I was nervous, but the reporter and cameraman were both really nice and put me at ease the whole time.

I had to wait forever for them to air the story though and I didn't know when they were going to run it. It was so funny when they finally did. I happened to be in the middle of a plank at my kickboxing class when one of the other ladies yelled out, "Shari!

You're on TV!" I don't think I have ever jumped up so quick in a training class!

I ran over to the TV to watch. It was so exciting to see myself on TV. The story was awesome and I really hoped it showed other people watching who struggle with their weight that it can be done and they CAN change their story just as I did.

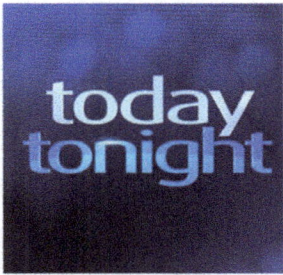

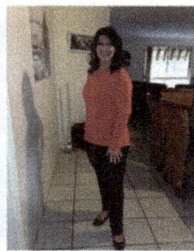

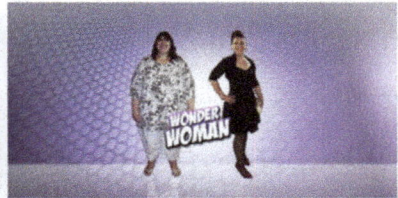

AU.NEWS.YAHOO.COM
Weight loss transformation – Today Tonight
A woman who used to weigh more than 180 kilogra...

After that, I also had That's Life and Take 5 magazines do stories on me.

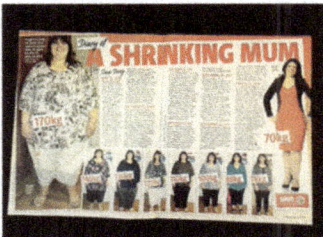

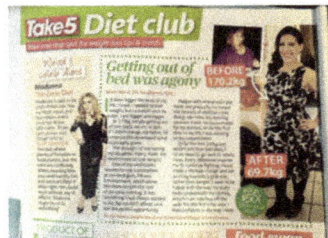

In February of 2013 I started my Personal Training course. It's forever in my mind that this is a lifetime commitment and I realized that I needed to do whatever I could to keep in the mindset of health and fitness, otherwise I could very easily find myself right back where I started. By becoming a Personal Trainer, I would continually be around like minded people and have to keep myself at a certain standard if I was to set a good example for my clients. I also wanted to help as many people as I could do what I have done, and becoming a Personal Trainer seemed like the perfect way to do that.

I also decided that it was time to start looking into excess skin removal surgery. I still had weight to release, but I couldn't tell what I still needed to work on because I had so much excess skin that no matter how much strengthening and toning exercise I did, I couldn't see any results.

I knew I would probably have to go overseas to have it done, but I did do my due diligence and had a consult with a surgeon on the Gold Coast to get a quote before I made the final decision. The day I went for the consult was an interesting process. The surgeon asked me how I had released the weight and I told him diet and exercise. He had a look at my excess skin and I gave him some blood results that my doctor had sent along with me for the consult.

Upon looking at them he smiled and said he could tell that I had released the weight naturally. I was curious to know how he could tell that and asked how he could. The surgeon explained that he quite often performed excess skin removal surgery on people who had weight loss surgery of various kinds, whether it be lap band or gastric sleeve, and it showed in their blood results. Our blood tells a story apparently and he said that while my blood results showed I had really good nutrition, quite often those of people that have had weight loss surgery show nutrition deficits because of the small amount of food they can actually eat.

Whilst I know some people who struggle with their weight feel their only option is to go down the path of bariatric surgery, I am so grateful that I managed to find my way to do it naturally and didn't have to go down that path.

Once I had the quote from the surgeon here and the quote from the overseas surgeon, I decided to go with the overseas option. The difference between the two quotes was $20,000. I already had to get a loan to have the surgery done in the first place and I also knew that I would probably have to get more done down the road as well, so Thailand it was.

I was lucky that I personally knew two people who had recently been over to Thailand to have surgery done and so I spoke to them and went with their recommendations from what they had both experienced personally. I applied for the loan, it was granted and I booked the first surgery for the 18th of August 2013. I would be having at least two surgeries while I was over there, but the exact date for the second one would be based on how I recovered from the first one.

I booked the first surgery and then booked my flights to give me enough time for at least 3 surgeries and a week to recuperate before I had to get back on a plane to fly home. I didn't know how I was going to make it all happen, but I was determined and with every step closer I got, I became more and more excited.

I had planned to go on my own. I wasn't going to ask anyone to go with me because it was a big financial expense. But I had come so far and fought so hard to get to this point that I wasn't going to let anything deter me. My family didn't want me to go overseas for the surgery and they didn't want me to go on my own, so in the end my mum decided to come with me. I didn't ask her to, but she volunteered and I was happy to have her come along.

Whilst I was making all my surgery arrangements, I had a call from Roula at The Biggest Loser Club. She had been contacted by Channel 9 Mornings about my story and she wanted to know if I would do an interview with them. Hellooooooo! There wasn't even a question of saying no! I told Roula that I would be going overseas for my surgery, but she said it wasn't a problem and she would coordinate a date for after I arrived back in Australia and recovered enough to travel down to Sydney for the interview.

Arriving in Bangkok on the evening of 17th August 2013, we were picked up and taken to the hospital where I would be having my surgery the next day. My mum and I would spend that night in the hospital apartment together and then my mum would remain in the hospital apartment until it was time for me to go to the hotel for recovery. On the morning of 18th of August 2013, I met with my surgeon and then waited until it was time for my surgery.

The first surgery was going to be my arms and breasts. I had massive bat wings of excess skin on my arms and my breasts were just 2 sacks of saggy skin hanging down to my belly button. I'm not exaggerating! I was so excited that I was finally going to get rid of all that saggy excess skin that I had absolutely no hesitation or concerns about any risk. I felt super fit, strong and healthy and had been sticking to a strict training and nutrition regime leading up to the surgery.

The final 6 weeks prior to the surgery in particular I was super focused on my training and nutrition so I would be as fit, healthy and strong as I could possibly be. I also had a friend who was a nurse who gave me some advice regarding certain supplements that I should take in the 6 weeks leading up to the surgery and 6 weeks after that would aid in my recovery. I felt nothing but total confidence!

The first surgery went well. Apparently I lost a lot of blood on the table, but otherwise everything was fine and I had 3 days recovery before I went to the hotel for the first time. One week after the first surgery I had my second surgery. This surgery was major and consisted of them cutting me right around my entire body - cutting out all the excess skin, pulling down from the top, pulling up from the bottom and sewing me back together. Pretty massive when you think about it. All I thought about was how wonderful it was going to be not to have all that saggy skin around the middle of my body anymore that I had to try and stuff into clothes!

My second surgery also went well. I did feel the impact of this one on my body more, which was to be expected. I was in a lot more pain and was much more uncomfortable, but I was prepared for it and it was definitely worth it. I stayed for 5 days in the hospital. It was good to have my mum there for moral support and I was also lucky she was there because she noticed an infection that had started that I couldn't see or feel. The nurses were giving me bed baths and missed that I was getting an infection where I had stitches right at the top of my butt crack. Lovely imagery I know, but if you're ever in this situation, it's better that you're aware of this stuff!

Before I left the hospital, I spoke to the surgeon about the surgery on my legs. When we had discussed it previously, he had said that he would see how the first 2 surgeries went and then we would talk about a further surgery. When I raised the topic with him again, he said that if I wanted him to, he would perform the surgery, but if it was him he would wait at least 6 months because it was too much of a risk at this point. Upon thinking about it, I decided I had fought so hard to get to this point, that it just wasn't worth the risk. If the surgeon was against it, then I should probably be safe rather than sorry and listen to his advice.

My mum and I went to the hotel for the rest of my recovery and it was at that point that I realized exactly how much impact the second surgery had on my body. In the hospital I had a raised hospital bed, but of course the bed in the hotel was flat and this is where I found that I REALLY needed my mum. I wasn't able to raise and lower myself, so if I didn't have my mum there, I wouldn't have been able to get in and out of bed. It was tough because it was hard for my mum to lift a dead weight up and down, but we managed somehow. I really don't know what I would have done without my mum!

Not long after I got to the hotel I decided that since I couldn't get my legs done, I should look into getting my teeth done, especially since I was going to be on tv again. So I called my surgery company liaison and asked if she could organize for me to have a quote done. I went in for the quote, was happy with it and organized to have porcelain veneers put on all the teeth that could be seen when I smiled. I had to have a total of 20 – 10 on the bottom and 10 on the top. I had it done in the last week of my recovery before I flew home and had absolutely beautiful perfect white teeth. I was so happy! I was still in pain but it was all so worth it and despite my pain and discomfort, I felt like a new person.

Monday the 9th of September was the day we were flying home. We checked out of the hotel and had to go to see the surgeon to have my stitches and staples removed as well as the last two drains that I still had attached to my wounds. I was a little worried because the surgeon had said that if the draining hadn't slowed to a certain point, then I would have to keep the drains in and he would remove them back home in Australia. I told him that I was NOT going to fly home with them attached to me. I knew the flight was going to be uncomfortable enough without me having to have two drains to worry about.

My final appointment with the surgeon was both good and bad. He agreed to remove the drains, but removing the staples was so painful. I felt every single staple come out and not in a good way. I don't think he cared about how much pain I was in and really just ripped them out one by one.

The flight home was extremely uncomfortable, but I made it through. I couldn't sit in my seat the whole time and spent quite a bit of time standing up. I tried to sleep but wasn't successful. When I got home and finally crawled into my own bed again I had the best sleep I'd had for a very, very long time.

My Channel 9 Mornings interview was scheduled for the 11th of October 2013. I flew down to Sydney on the 10th and stayed in a hotel overnight because I had to be at the Channel 9 studios early for hair and makeup before the interview. Roula came to the hotel in a cab to pick me up and we travelled to the studio together. She stayed with me the whole time while I was getting my hair and makeup done. Have I mentioned how much I love having my hair and makeup done?! I felt like such a star!

What was even more exciting – I know, I know – how can this possibly get even more exciting? Well it did, because while I was getting my hair done, Karl Stefanovic stuck his head in and spoke to the lady doing my hair. He looked at me as if he was trying to figure out who I was, smiled at me and then went on his way down the hallway. After my hair had been done I had to go down the hallway to another room to have my makeup done. While a lady was doing my face, guess who came in to have makeup done as well? Rob Mills! Australian Idol contestant, Winners & Losers, Young Talent Time. Anyway... he came in, took his shirt off right beside me, sat in the other makeup chair and asked if someone could do his face. I was in heaven! At one point he smiled at me and said something to the effect that I didn't need makeup. I don't quite remember exactly what he said, because I couldn't really think properly!

From there it all seemed like a bit of a whirlwind. Makeup was finished and I was taken over to where I had to wait my turn to be interviewed. I was being interviewed by David Campbell and Livinia Nixon. I was so nervous! It was live tv and I was so worried I was going to be too nervous to talk or get tongue tied or say something really stupid. The interview I did for Today Tonight could be edited, this couldn't be.

Finally it was my turn and it was so bright under those lights. I had a really tall stool to sit on and I was scared I was going to catch my heel on it and fall off. The interview was over in a flash but I felt it went really well. Roula was so excited when I got back to her. She said I looked great, spoke really well and called me a super star.

Every now and then I rewatch that interview and the excitement of my five minutes of fame comes rushing back every single time!

Roula and I made our way back to the foyer to wait for a taxi and guess who we saw talking to someone in the carpark while we were waiting? The handsome Rob Mills again! Roula was watching me and laughingly encouraged me to go and ask him for a photo. It was obvious that I wanted to, but I was too shy to ask. Finally I got up the courage and he happily agreed. He asked what my interview had been about and I told him and he gave me a high 5. I thought that was the end of it, but then he said he'd noticed we had been waiting there for a while and asked what we were waiting for. We told him we were waiting for a taxi. He then asked where we needed to go and Roula told him. Then, Rob Mills offered to give us a ride! Oh my goodness! I could hardly believe it! Of course we said yes!

We talked the whole way about Grease, which was the musical he was currently performing in amongst other things. I seriously did not want it to end. Unfortunately we eventually arrived at our destination and we hopped out. He was a real gentleman and got my carry on suitcase out of the car and put it on the footpath beside me. Then he gave me a kiss on the cheek before he left. I must've been bright red. Roula laughed and told me he had obviously taken a real shine to me. She hailed a cab, helped me into it and waved as I continued onto the airport to fly home. It was an amazing day. I'm sure he probably wouldn't remember a scrap of it, but for me it was another day that will be forever etched into my memory.

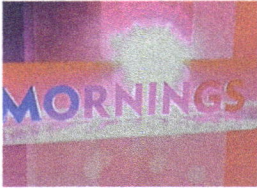

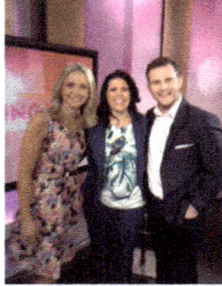

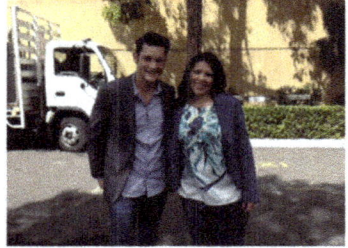

You can watch part of the interview at: http://bit.ly/2v2jAld

The rest of 2013 was spent helping my daughter organize her impending trip to the US, where she was going to spend a year or so with family and go to college. We enjoyed a lovely Christmas together which we knew could be the last one for a while and then came New Year, which I spent carrying out my annual ritual. I once again celebrated the New Year and spent New Year's Day reflecting on the year, making goals for the year ahead.

On the 8th of January 2014 I drove my beautiful daughter to the airport and bid a teary farewell as she boarded the plane for the first leg of her trip to the US for an undetermined period of time. I knew that I would miss her greatly. We are very close my girl and I.

We'd never spent longer than 6 weeks apart and that was only once in her 18 years. Whilst I would miss her though, I was excited for her going off on her own adventure out into the big wide world and I was also excited to be beginning my own adventure completely on my own. I knew there were exciting times ahead for both of us!

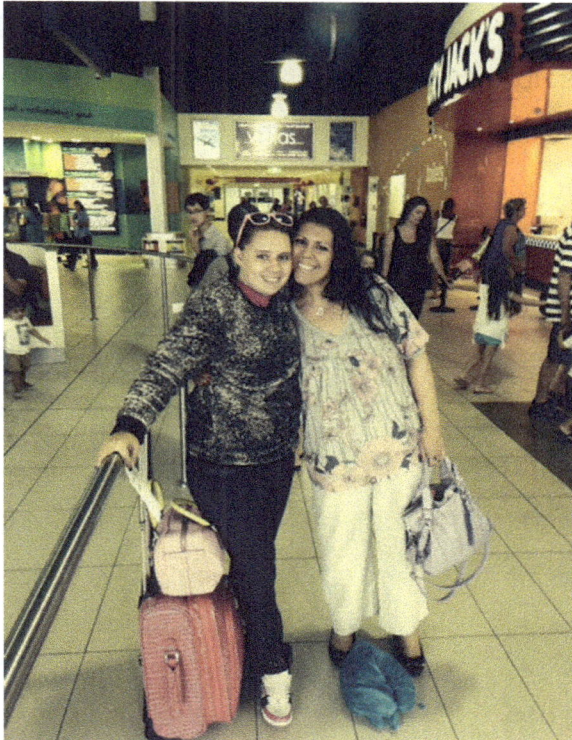

Saying goodbye to my girl!!

On the 21st of January 2014 I had my final surgery to date – my legs. I had them done here in Australia on the Gold Coast where

I live. They cut a big V shaped wedge out of the inside of each leg, pulled the edges back in together and stitched them up. I have scars right down the inside of my legs and the inside of my groin on both sides. I was in hospital initially until the 27th of January and was allowed to go home to continue recovering on the proviso that I kept my legs up.

What I didn't realize though, was that when the surgeon said to keep my legs up – he actually meant UP! I figured that sitting at a desk with my feet slightly elevated all day while I worked was enough, but obviously not. It was also the height of summer and I had no air conditioning where I lived, only fans, so the combination of the heat and not having my legs elevated enough both contributed to me getting an infection. The surgeon shook his head at me and readmitted me to hospital on the 3rd of February where I stayed for another week or so. I wasn't allowed to go home until the surgeon was satisfied that the infection was under control. He also made me it very clear that for the next few weeks I was to be confined to my bed with my legs completely UP.

I worked that way for weeks until the surgeon gave me the all clear to do otherwise. Those first few weeks recovering at home were interesting to say the least. I have to say that I didn't realize that the position of my "who-ha" would change as a result of the surgery. I had to learn to pee all over again and I had quite a few accidents. I actually kept a mop and bucket in the toilet for a while because it was that frequent. This may be TMI for some, but if you're considering surgery such as this, it's better to be forewarned. My surgeon didn't think to mention it, so the first time I went to the toilet after my surgery I made a right royal mess and had no idea what the heck was going on!

The rest of 2014 was mostly spent finishing off my Personal Training qualification and starting to set up my new personal training business. In November of 2014 I also decided that it was time for me to write my story. It took me 3 years to write it. There's a whole other story in that, which we'll get to later on.

The year 2015 dawned and it was my first year of fitness challenges, beginning with the Q1 Stair Challenge on the Gold Coast where I live in February. The Q1 has 77 flights of stairs that we had to run up. It took me just over 19 minutes – the LONGEST 19 minutes of my life. I didn't run the whole way, but I didn't stop either, so I was proud of myself.

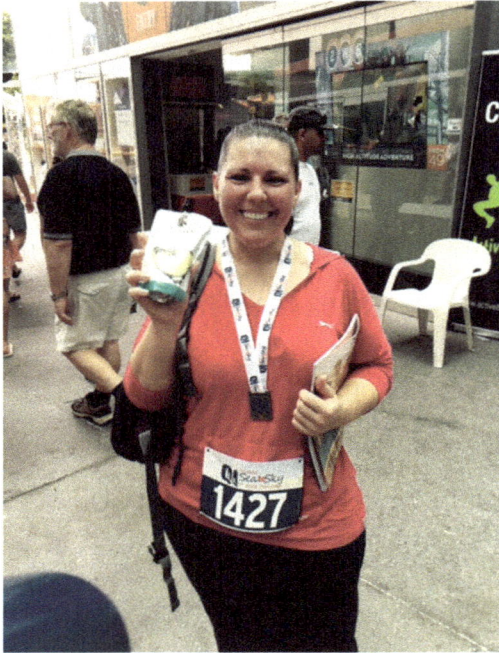

Q1 Stair Challenge!

Once I had completed that challenge, I set my sights on my next one. A few years before, when I was near the beginning of my weight release journey, I had set myself the goal of doing the 10km run in the Gold Coast Marathon. I trained for it, but I was still very overweight and I knew that I couldn't finish in the time allotted so I didn't register for it. In 2015 I decided it was time for me to set myself another running goal, and since I knew I could run 10km already as I had done so as part of my training regime in recent times, there was no point doing that. I didn't see the point in paying money to do something that I had already done.

So I decided that if I was going to challenge myself, I had to do the half marathon, because I sure was NOT going to even consider doing a full marathon. That's for crazy people! I'm also not a runner. I run slower than a herd of elephants stampeding through peanut butter and I'm not exaggerating even a tiny bit! I do not look in any way elegant or attractive when I run and I really don't like it. I was worried that I wouldn't make the cut off and get my medal because I struggled to run at a fast enough pace throughout my training leading up to it.

In the midst of my training, I enjoyed a very special birthday. On Saturday the 13th of June I turned 40. I had been so looking forward to my 40th birthday. I had a whole new amazing world in front of me and it felt like my 40th was the entrance to it. My debut into it, so to speak. The theme of my birthday party was "Dreams Do Come True" – my dreams certainly did and they're still coming true to this day, one by one. I bought a beautiful dress for the occasion and accessories to match. I had my hair and makeup done and I looked and felt like a princess. I enjoyed my night immensely and then got my head back in the game for the upcoming half marathon.

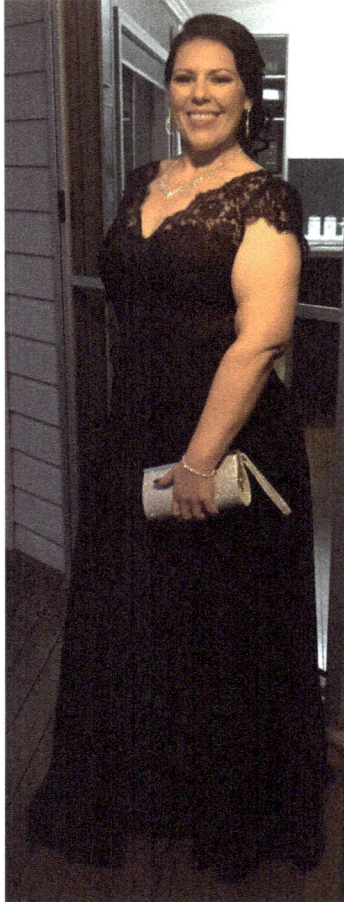

My 40th birthday!

On Sunday 5th July 2015 I set off on my first massive physical fitness challenge. I knew it would take me at least 3 hours if not longer and I had 3 hours and 20 minutes if I wanted to get my medal. I definitely wanted to get my medal! I crossed the finish line in just under 3 hours, which totally blew me away! I got my shiny medal, but the year wasn't done just yet...

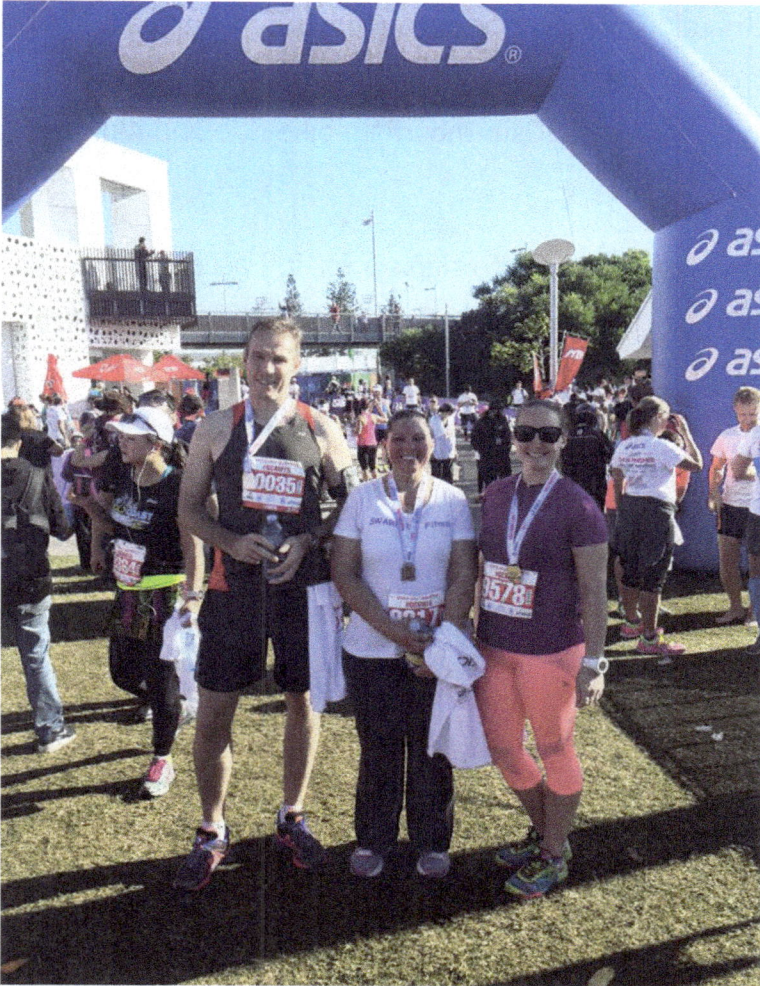

21.1km done!

A lady by the name of Lyndell with a similar weight release story had found me through Facebook. We had met in person to talk about our experiences and became good friends. Lyndell worked for a company that ran what's called an Adventurethon which is like a triathlon, but over ocean and trails, not the road. They had an event called the "Taste of Adventurethon", which consisted of a 1km ocean paddle, 10km mountain bike ride and 4km trail/beach run.

Lyndell encouraged me to sign up for it. I accepted the challenge, even though I knew it would be WAY out of my comfort zone. Luckily, the house I was renting at the time backed onto a creek that flowed out into the Broadwater and my house was only about 250 meters away from the mouth. The owners had a kayak they had left behind with the house and had said I could use it if I wanted. It came in very handy I can tell you.

The first time I went for a paddle I ended up swimming... twice... and found out after the fact that there have been sightings of bull sharks in that creek....yikes! My paddling got better over time until I finally felt courageous enough to paddle out in the actual Broadwater. I only managed to do that a couple of times before the actual event.

On Saturday the 12th of October I travelled down to Coffs Harbour with a friend who was going to help me with my change overs and my gear. The event was being held on the Sunday morning, so we travelled down on Saturday and stayed overnight. On Sunday 13th of October we drove to the event site, set up all my gear and I lined up with the rest of the competitors.

The starting gun went off and we had a short run down to the beach to our kayaks. We had to drag our kayaks into the water and paddle out into the ocean 500 metres, navigate around a couple of buoys to get back to shore and complete a total distance of 1km. The sea that day was very choppy and I wasn't experienced enough. I ended up getting dumped unceremoniously about 5 metres out and had to follow my kayak back to shore. Luckily a lovely spectator had seen what happened and came to hold the kayak for me while I got back on. That 1km paddle was seriously one of the scariest things I have ever done in my life. I knew that if I tipped over out in the open water, I probably wouldn't be able to get back into my kayak and wouldn't be able to finish. The thought of drowning did cross my mind, although I float pretty well and I was also wearing a life jacket, so it was really only an issue in my head!

The whole time I was paddling, I kept saying over and over, "Slow and steady wins the race. I can do this. Everything is going to be ok. Please keep me safe Dad!" Over and over and over. I didn't stop chanting until I got back to shore safe and sound. I pulled my kayak back onto the shore, heaved a massive sigh of relief and set off running up to the bike area. I made up some time I had lost on the bike leg, despite crashing at one point!

The run was the final leg and while most of it was ok, there was one part where we had to edge our way along a very narrow path with a very sheer drop down the side of a cliff on one side. I just kept telling myself I would be fine and asking my Dad to keep me safe. I felt so relieved, happy and proud to cross the finish line that day I can tell you.

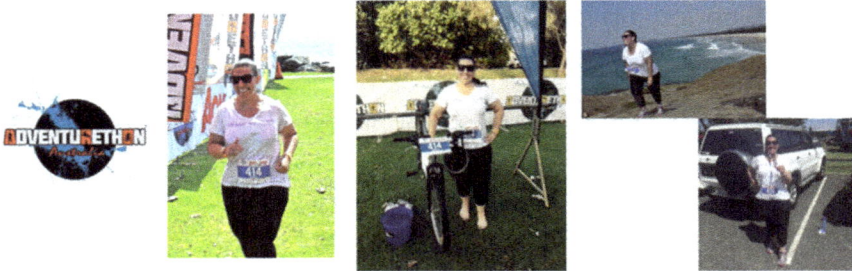

I then ended the year with a bang! On the 10th of December 2015 I departed on a flight to the US to surprise my daughter for Christmas. I hadn't seen her for almost two years and while I had had some amazing adventures, I had missed her so much. She was coming home just after Christmas, but what she didn't know was that I was coming to spend Christmas with her and our family over there and that we would fly home together in time for New Year. We had a wonderful, picture perfect white Christmas, just as I had hoped and made some wonderful memories before we came back home together.

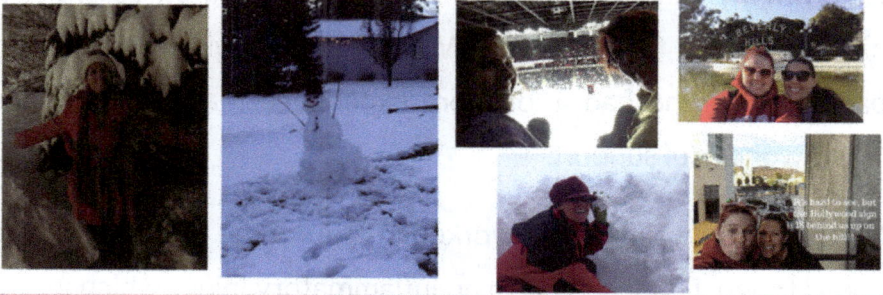

Although the years prior to 2016 were massive, I knew even before it started that 2016 was going to be a monumental year and what a year it was! Once again on New Year's Day I sat down – this time with my daughter – and we both wrote down our New Year's Resolutions.

I had several New Year's resolutions, just as I do every year. I'm a continual work in progress in so many areas of my life; relationships, work, health & fitness, financial. I had a couple of massive physical challenges on my list - I had some crazy idea that I could run my first marathon (and most probably my only marathon!) and 2 weeks later complete the Kokoda Challenge which is 96km of trekking through the Gold Coast Hinterland – up and down a LOT of mountains! Just to make it even more interesting, in between those two events was my daughter's 21st birthday. Wow! It made me feel exhausted just thinking about it!

Training for both the marathon and the Kokoda Challenge began in January. Marathon training was on my own, whilst Kokoda training was with my daughter and our two other team mates. You have to have a team of four to enter. We also trained with another team participating who had a lot more experience that we did, which was a wonderful support.

My marathon training was worked in around the Kokoda training. It was tough. I ended up with an inflammatory injury which wasn't going to resolve until I stopped running, if at all. I refused to give in. I also had a knee injury at one point. I rested when I needed to, had regular allied professional visits to manage the injuries and I listened to my body. I did my best, but I didn't get to where I wanted to in my training before the marathon and I was still too slow. I had 6 hours and 40 minutes and once again, I didn't know if I would make the cutoff and get my shiny medal.

Sunday the 3rd of July arrived and I rocked up to the starting line having made the decision that no matter what had happened during my training, I had paid for it and I was going to do my best. I was NOT going to give up without a fight. I also decided that this time, I was going to enjoy the experience as much as I could, despite the bit about running for over 6 hours!

The starting gun went off and we were on our way. My pace was better than it had ever been in training. At every checkpoint I was ahead of time. I had fun with it. I high fived spectators along the way. I joked with people holding supportive signs for us. I asked people at coffee shops to order me a full fat caramel latte and run it up the road to me. I didn't run very fast so they would definitely be able to catch me I told them! I asked the police lady to arrest me so I didn't have to keep running. I asked the ambos what I had to do to get a ride to the finish line.

I slowed down... YES... even I was amazed that I actually had to slow down at times to give moral support to other runners that were struggling and looking like they wanted to give up. I told them my story and they could do whatever they told themselves they could and that they just needed to believe in themselves, and they smiled and kept going. I found my daughter at the 32km mark waiting to give me a hug and I told her how strong I still felt.

At about 35kms I hit the wall. I'd been told about it. I was hoping I wouldn't hit it, but I did. It was good that I hit it there though, because I only had 7km to go. I had already run 35kms and I was well ahead of time. I told myself that even if I slowed down, as long as I kept going I would make it and get my shiny medal. I wanted that shiny medal so bad! I had come this far and I was *not* going to give up.

The whole rest of the way I kept chanting, "Slow and steady wins the race, one step at a time, you can do this, I am going to get that shiny medal!" I kept chanting over and over in my head. I definitely slowed down, but I refused to stop running. I finally got to the "250m to go" sign, ran under it and around the corner, found my daughter along the fence waiting for me and ran over to her. I hugged her tight because I knew that not only would I cross that finish line, but I would do it in time to get my medal. I was laughing and crying as I hugged her and told her I would see her on the other side. Then I continued to cross the finish line in 6 hours and 19 minutes. Words simply cannot describe how I felt when I crossed that line. I did a video when I got home. You can watch the video at: https://youtu.be/id-2mFvJTOs.

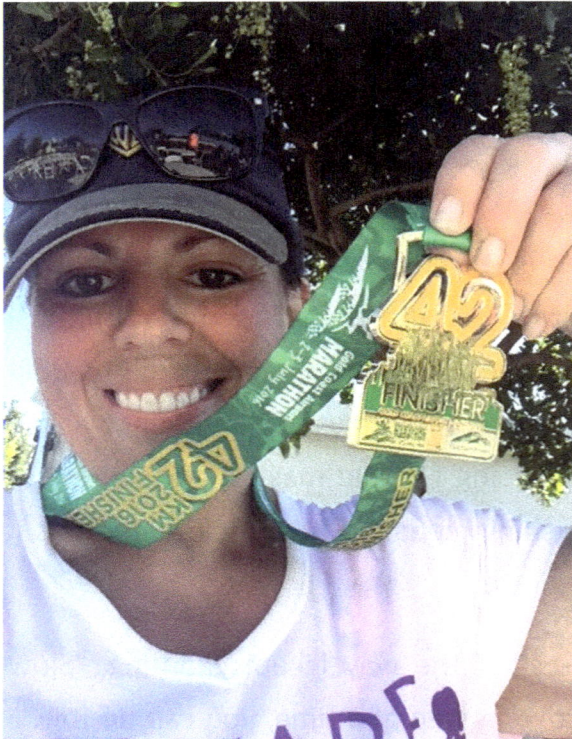

I got my shiny medal!

The following week was my daughter's 21st birthday. It was a wonderful evening spent with family and friends and definitely a highlight of our year.

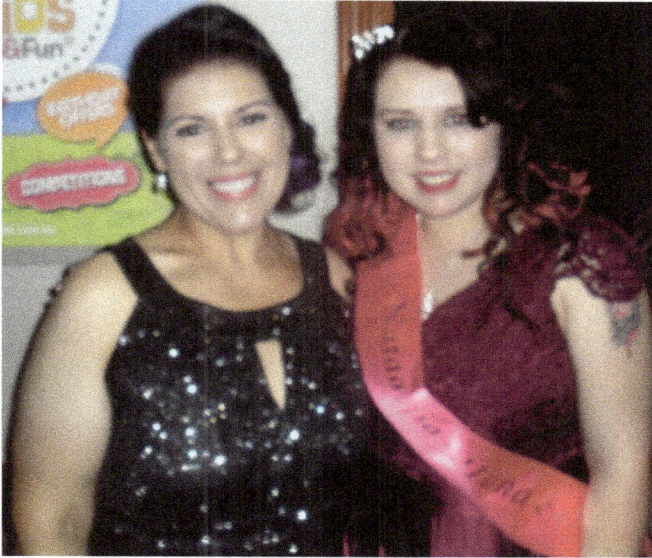

A week later, it was Kokoda Challenge time. Unfortunately, we weren't able to complete it. We managed to trek 43.2km, but had to pull out at that point because we had two team members who were in too much pain to continue. I jokingly say that at least I got 1km further than my marathon! We will attempt the Kokoda Challenge again in the future. I like to finish what I start. Sometimes it takes me a while, but I always finish in the end.

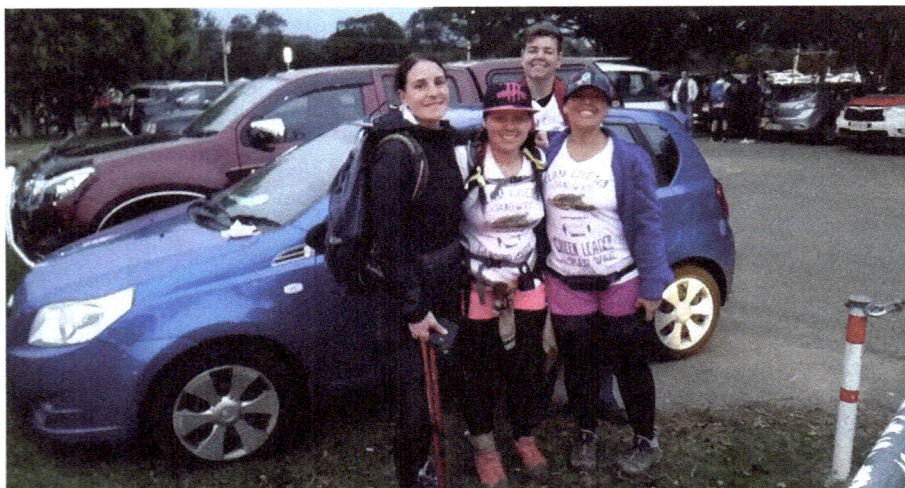

Our Kokoda Challenge team – Team Chicken Sandwich!

I want to make it clear that I couldn't have achieved or even wanted to achieve all that I have if I hadn't successfully released the weight. With every kilo that I released, I became more confident and more willing to get out of my comfort zone. The more I tested the waters and challenged myself and succeeded, the stronger my self belief became. It didn't happen overnight, but it did happen. Like a butterfly emerging from a cocoon.

2017 was an eventful year. I started out the year with my normal New Year routine and I slowly but surely worked on the goals that I set for myself. One of the most notable events of the year was attending a Hypnosis Certification Course in February which set me on a path of further personal development. In September 2017, I had the opportunity to attend a Tony Robbins event with my daughter and her partner which began with walking on fire!

Through the Hypnosis Course I was given the opportunity to sign up for an NLP (Neuro Linguistic Programming) Certification Course. The 13th of October seems to be a good day for me because on that day in 2017 I began my NLP course and my world expanded even more. The course was split into two phases and I learned and grew so much in such a short period of time. Not only am I a fire walker, but during the NLP course I had the opportunity to eat fire and break a wooden board with my bare hand and I succeeded at both of them.

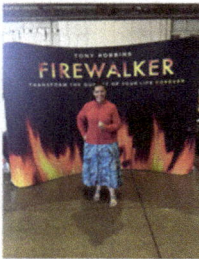

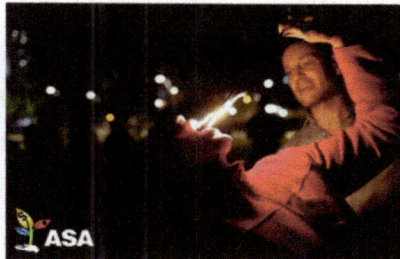

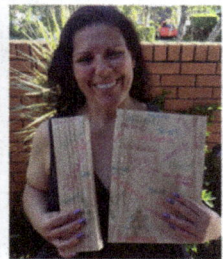

My list of credentials is ever increasing and I have no plans to slow down. I now have many more tools in my tool kit to help those that struggle with their weight as I used to and I feel so blessed to be able to help people change their story as I have done.

There was one other notable achievement for 2017 and that was that I finished writing this book. I started to write this book 3 years ago on November 2nd 2014. Why did it take me so long? Definitely not because it was so difficult or lengthy or anything like that. It was all about fear. It had been almost finished for the last three years. I decided that I was going to finish it during November of 2017, and that's what I did. In one month, I finished the first draft and also did my first edit. That's something that I had been trying to do for 3 years and the reason why I struggled with it is because of what would happen after it was finished.

After it was finished, it would then be published. Then what would happen? People would read it of course! Then what would happen? What would people think? What would my family think? There is some personal stuff in here. It's embarrassing. Will people judge me? Will they look at me different? Do you see how the subconscious mind can either help or hinder you when you are trying to achieve a goal? Through the power of NLP, I no longer let those fears hold me back. Now all I think about is who will it help? If my story and the things I've learned and am passing on help just one person, then it's totally worth it.

Another one of my big goals is my final body goal. When I talk about my goal body, it's hard to put a number of any kind on it. People quite often ask me what my goal weight is, and while I can say a number, it's really only an estimation because I actually don't know what my end weight will be. My actual goal is what I want my body to look like. Don't get me wrong, I absolutely love my body and so I should! It's put up with such bad treatment from me and it just keeps going and going and going! I have come so far and I have this amazing life now which I absolutely

LOVE, but I am always looking for ways to improve and this is one of them. I have absolutely no doubt that I will reach my goal. If there is one thing that I have learned over my journey, it's that absolutely ANYTHING is possible if your why is strong enough. In the meantime though, I am so very happy, healthy, fit and strong!

My business and financial goals are tied in together. I decided that I was going to head off in a different direction with my fitness business. I realized that I needed to go more in the direction of face to face and online weight release programs and support, rather than physically personal training with people. I am so glad that I became qualified as a personal trainer. It's something that I will always use to help the people that I help, but I stopped and thought about it a bit more and realised that the people I really want to help and come to me for help are those that are very overweight. Exercise is the last piece of the puzzle for them. I certainly didn't start with exercise. Exercise was the last thing I added in after I had sorted out my head and started eating right and that's how I help people now.

As I have said before, the first step is to address what's going on in our head, the second step is to change the way we eat and then after we've got those two things under control, we start to add in exercise and make other changes we know we need to make. A lot of people I help are not at the point of starting to exercise for a very long time and of course I am able to help them when they get to that point, but it's not where we start.

I start by helping people change their mindset, and by moving my business online, I have been able to help so many more people. I want to get to the end of my life (which is years and years and years away!) knowing that I have helped thousands of people change their lives and become happier, healthier and fitter just like I have. I'm doing that by using all the amazing tools I have in my tool belt such as Hypnotherapy and NLP, Personal Training and my own personal journey to mentor people on their own journey from Fat to FABulous. I work with people on an individual basis to make the necessary changes one at a time and in a way that they can not only release the weight, but keep it off for life. So that they create a life they LOVE!

SHARI'S FAB SECRET KEY TO SUCCESS

Belief is imperative. You CAN do ANYTHING you tell yourself you can! If you want to successfully release your weight, you must firstly believe that it's possible and secondly you must believe in yourself and your ability to make the changes that you need to make!

"The body achieves what the mind believes" ~ Author unknown

Chapter Four

Your Fat to Fabulous Keys to Success

So... What does this all mean for you? How can you do what I've done? Because you can! I'm just a normal person like you. The only difference is I figured out what was going on in my subconscious and worked with it to get the results I wanted.

I read an awesome book called, *The Secret Code of Success* by Noah St John. It explained what happened to me so well, I now use it to explain it to others. In the book Noah says, "You can't fix a Why To problem with a How To answer."

What this means is we all *know* how to release weight. We know that we need to eat better and add in some exercise if we can. So why don't we do it? We don't do it because our reasons why we *want* to are not strong enough to override all the reasons why we *don't* want to.

We know HOW to lose weight, but because our reasons why we don't want to are bigger than our reasons why we do want to, we don't. If I had a $1 for every time someone has asked me what the secret is, I would be a millionaire. There really is no secret other than you need to make your reasons WHY you want to release the weight greater than all your reasons you DON'T want to.

When you do this, you'll be able to achieve whatever goal you have set for yourself and it won't seem nearly as hard as you thought it would, because you want it so much. You CAN do whatever you tell yourself you can, if you want to badly enough.

So let's get started!

KEY 1: Your WHY

The first thing you need to do is take some time out to concentrate on yourself. Start a list of reasons why you want to release weight and a list of reasons why you don't want to. I know this sounds silly, but it's really important. This process may take some time, so start your list and keep it handy, so that over the coming days or weeks, you can add to it whenever something pops into your head.

Once you start consciously thinking about something, your subconscious will keep it ticking over and things will just occur to you out of the blue, so it's important to write them down as they do so you don't forget them. I cannot stress enough how important this first part of the process is.

When it comes to reasons why, it should be pretty easy. There are many reasons why you might want to release weight. To be healthier, to live longer, to fit into nicer clothes, to feel better, to be able to do things with your loved ones, to lead a good example for your children and I know there are many more we could all come up with.

This is the easy part of the process, but make sure you write down as many as you possibly can - you will need every single one of them in your arsenal!

The hard part, and the most important part of this first step in the process, is to write your list of why you DON'T want to. This is where you need to be honest with yourself. There are lots of conscious reasons why we don't want to release weight. I'll give you some examples so you understand how honest you need to be and that you can put anything on the list, no matter how ridiculous or stupid you may think it is.

One of my clients asked me if a reason why not to release weight could be they just loved yummy food too much and didn't want to give it up. My answer was of course it's a reason why not! It may seem stupid to put things like that on your list, but if it's something that applies to you, then it's a reason why you're not making the changes you need to make.

Other reasons could be it's too hard, you don't have enough time, you're too tired... Be honest, really think about it and if it's something that seems valid for you, then it needs to go on the list so it can be addressed.

This is also the part of the process where you need to dig right down inside yourself, analyse yourself, your behaviour and your triggers. Try to think about things you do to sabotage your efforts and why you might do them. This will help you identify some of the more unconscious reasons why you might not want to release weight.

Quite often it's stuff that's happened in our past that can be a really big reason why we don't want to release weight. But when we're able to identify it, it's easier to address it. As I have said previously, my biggest reason why I didn't want to release weight was because I didn't want to have a relationship. I didn't want to be attractive to the opposite sex and being overweight was my way of making myself so unattractive that I didn't have to worry about it. It was my suit of armour to keep my heart protected, because I had been hurt in my previous relationships. Absolutely ridiculous I know. For a long time I didn't even realise that's what I was doing and when I eventually did realise it, it still wasn't something I was able to overcome, until it was no longer a reason for me to stay overweight.

I was only finally able to successfully release the weight because I no longer wanted to be single. I didn't want to be alone for the rest of my life, sitting on the couch watching tv. I wanted to find someone to share my life with and I wanted that so much I was able to do what I needed to do to release the weight.

This is why this step in the process is so, so important! If your reasons WHY are strong enough to outweigh the WHY NOT reasons you have, you're going to be successful at whatever you try to achieve.

Focus on your WHY – what you focus on is what you get!

SHARI'S FAB ACTION STEP

Get yourself a special book which you can call your FAB planner and a pen, draw a line down the middle of the front page, write WHY's on the left at the top and WHY NOT's on the right and start writing down your reasons for each side.

KEY 2: Belief

The second most important thing is having belief. Firstly, you need to believe what you're trying to achieve is possible in the first place, otherwise, why would you even try? Secondly, you absolutely have to believe in yourself. You have to know that you are enough. That you are worthy. That you CAN do anything you tell yourself you can.

What you focus on is what you get, so focus on the belief that you CAN change your story, one step at a time and you'll find that's exactly what happens.

We all have limiting beliefs. We tell ourselves lots of stories like, "I have bad genes", "It's too hard to eat healthy", "I'm too lazy to exercise", "I'm too old to change my ways now", "I can't do it". Do any of these sound familiar to you? They're all limiting beliefs and when you substitute empowering beliefs in their place, such as "I CAN do it!", you will be amazed at how much easier the process becomes.

I had so many limiting beliefs! One of the biggest ones was that eating certain foods would automatically make me gain weight. Another was that I wasn't important. I know I definitely had the limiting belief of having bad genes! There were many, many more and it would take me all day to list them, but you get the idea. I have overcome a lot of limiting beliefs on my journey and it's something I work on on a daily basis.

SHARI'S FAB ACTION STEP

Get out your FAB planner and a red and a green pen. Write a list of your own limiting beliefs in red, with a couple of lines in between each of them. Once you've done that, get the green pen, draw a line through the first limiting belief (crossing it out) and write an empowering belief underneath it. Do the same for each limiting belief you have written down. For example, if you have written, "It's hard to eat healthy", cross it out with the green pen and write underneath it something like, "It's easy to eat healthy because it makes me feel so good!"

KEY 3: Goal

The next step in the process is to set yourself a goal and it needs to be a SMART goal. I know, I know… we've all heard it before… but it works and I use this process regularly in my life for every single goal that I have.

A SMART goal stands for Specific, Measureable, Achievable, Realistic, Timeframe. So don't just write down that you need to release weight. How much weight? Is it a weight goal or is it a health goal? Do you want to fit into a certain pair of jeans? Or do you want to be able to walk up a set of stairs without collapsing at the top? It needs to be important to YOU.

Whatever it is, be Specific about exactly what it is. Make sure it can be Measured and write down how. Make sure that it's Achievable and Realistic. For example, don't make your goal that you want to lose 10kg in 2 weeks. If it's not achievable and realistic, you're setting yourself up for disappointment right from the get go. Lastly, make sure you decide on a Timeframe, which obviously needs to be achievable and realistic as well.

The second year of my weight release journey was the year I knew I needed to up the ante if I didn't want the process to take 10 years. So my goal for that year was:

- Specific: To get to double digits on the scale

- Measureable: I had to lose 60kgs

- Achievable: It worked out to be just over 1kg per week, so I felt it was achievable. Not easy, but achievable

- Realistic: Just over 1kg per week was realistic with the amount of weight I had to release. The heavier you are the better your results in the beginning usually are

- Timeframe: The deadline I set for myself was New Year's Eve 2011

Writing out your goals like this really helps you to get clear about where you're going and how you're going to get there.

SHARI'S FAB ACTION STEP

Get out your FAB planner and write down your goals in the above format. If you have more than 2, then pick 2 to focus on for the next 30 days and then reassess at the end of the 30 day period.

KEY 4: Vision

Once you've set your goal, take time out to envision your life when you achieve your goal. Some find it hard to keep motivated on the seemingly never ending journey of releasing weight and creating a healthier lifestyle. One of the things I encourage my clients to do is to envision what their life will be like when they get to their end goal.

It helps to sit down and write down some ways that your life will be different. What will you be able to do that you can't do now? How will your life change? How will you feel? Take some time out every day to sit with these things. Write a scenario about something you'll do when you get to your goal that you can't or don't want to do now because of your weight.

Every day, close your eyes for a few minutes and run through that scenario in your mind. Add to it. Make it better. Make it clearer. I do this every morning when I get up and every evening before I go to bed. The clearer your vision is and the more you keep it in mind, the easier it will be to get through the tough times. That vision is the reason you're doing the hard yards. It will all be worth the hard work in the end! Ask yourself, how will your life change when you get to your goal?

My initial vision was to be a normal size. To be able to fit into a chair with arms comfortably. To be able to do up the seat belt on an airplane. To be able to walk into a clothes store and choose something off the rack and it fit and actually look nice. I would sit and close my eyes and smile, picturing the exact scenarios in my mind. I would actually picture myself doing up the seat belt on the airplane and it fitting for the first time. I pictured myself walking into a clothing store and browsing and then walking to the change room and trying on whatever item I had chosen and it looking amazing on me!

SHARI'S FAB ACTION STEP

Get out your FAB planner and write down your vision. Make it something that makes your heart sing! Make it something that brings tears of joy to your eyes when you envision yourself achieving it. Make it as real as possible. Put in as much detail as possible. When you have written it out, close your eyes and run through the scenario in your head. Every little detail. Feel how it feels to have accomplished that. Smile and laugh and savour that feeling. Do this on a daily basis.

KEY 5: Strategy

Albert Einstein hit the nail on the head with his famous quote, "The definition of insanity is doing the same thing over and over again and expecting different results". And it's especially true when it comes to weight release.

If you've stuck at something consistently and you're not getting results, then nothing is going to change unless you change what you're doing. I know it sounds like a no brainer, but we all know that sometimes we keep doing the same thing time and time again and hope to get different results.

Unfortunately, it's not like your body is finally going to get the memo and jump on board with what your brain wants and start to toe the line. It doesn't mean that the method you're trying doesn't work – it just means that it doesn't work for YOU. If you want to change that, you need to do something different. You need a different strategy. You need to make changes, and that's the next step in the process.

I remember one time I was so desperate to release weight that I decided to try the modifast shakes. I persevered for a week and then I just couldn't do it any longer. They actually made me feel sick. I didn't like the taste of them and I really hated not eating real food. While I did release some weight while I was on them, I didn't feel that I could keep doing that long term and so I changed my strategy.

SHARI'S FAB ACTION STEP

Get out your FAB planner and write down any strategies to do with releasing weight that you've used in the past. Then tick them if they worked for you at the time and cross out any that didn't. Once you have done that, think about each of them in turn and see if you can identify why they worked or why they didn't. This will help you to come up with a strategy that will work better for you.

KEY 6: Change One Thing at A Time

If you have a weight issue, you'd probably agree that you need to make changes to your eating and exercise regime at the very least. Therefore, your next step is to write your list of all the things you need to change in order to reach your goal.

This might be a short list or it may be a long list. If your list is long, don't let yourself be overwhelmed or discouraged by it. You won't be trying to change everything at once. Just concentrate on writing your list. Make sure you're honest with yourself and put anything and everything on there that YOU feel you need or want to change to achieve your goal.

Once again, this may take some time and you should keep it handy so you can add to it whenever something pops into you head. Once you have your list of things you need to change, we're ready to get started.

Are you ready? Of course you are! You need to pick ONE thing off your list. Only one. That's what you're going to work on until you've made it a habit.

For example, if one of your things was to eat more vegetables, then for the next week, I want you to concentrate on eating more vegetables. You need to figure out how you're going to do that, make a plan and concentrate on putting it into action.

You won't try to change anything else until you're confident you have that under control. It doesn't matter what it is you choose first, but whatever you choose first should be something you feel you can definitely do without too much trouble. That way, when you achieve it, you'll feel so much happier with yourself and that will give you the confidence you need to make the next change you decide to make.

I tell my clients not to try to change too much at once, because when you try to do that, you become overwhelmed, it becomes way too hard and you end up throwing in the towel. Sound like a familiar scenario? Once you're positive that this change has become a habit, then choose the next thing you're going to change, make that a habit and then choose the next thing.

Yes, this will take time. It doesn't matter. By giving yourself time to make the changes into habits, you're giving yourself the best chance to not only release the weight, but to keep it off for the long term. It didn't take you 5 minutes to put it on, and it won't take 5 minutes to release it either. Slow and steady definitely wins the race when it comes to weight release.

One of my favourite ways to describe this is a saying that makes me giggle, but it's oh so true: "How do you eat an elephant? One bite at a time of course!" Releasing weight and creating a healthier lifestyle should be treated in exactly the same way. Sometimes it can seem like an insurmountable feat, but if you approach the problem in the right way, then you will make a lot more progress.

That's it. It's that simple. It really is. Your whole weight release journey will be one of deciding on the change that you're making next, implementing it, being consistent with it until it has become a habit and then moving onto the next one. Your why, your self belief and your vision will be the fuel that keeps you moving toward your goal at whatever pace is perfect for you.

Whilst the basic process is simple, there are a lot of tips that I have learned over the course of my own journey that made my journey quicker and easier and that will also help you along the way. In the following pages, I am going to impart the most important things I have learned over my journey thus far. They're all things you will implement over time, keeping to the premise of making one change at a time.

One of the biggest things that I've learned is the learning never EVER stops. There are always new things to learn, better ways of doing things and the first step is being open to that. The moment we think we've learned everything there is to learn, we're doing ourselves the biggest disservice. Just remember you don't need to try to make too many changes at once. I know I sound like a broken record, but I cannot say it enough... One change at a time!

SHARI'S FAB ACTION STEP

Get out your FAB planner and write down your list of things that you feel you need to change. Pick one thing, make a plan of action of how you're going to do that and get started. You CAN do it!

KEY 7: Break Your Goal Down into Mini Goals

I've said it before and I'll say it again... How do you eat an elephant? One bite at a time of course! If you have a lot of weight to release, it can be easy to become discouraged. While you certainly need to have a goal that you want to get to, the best way to tackle it is to break that end goal into smaller goals. I guess you could call them smaller, bite size chunks!

If I continually thought about the fact that I had at least 100kg to release, I would've been very discouraged! Instead I concentrated on releasing 10kg at a time. When I released 10kg, I had my photo taken, celebrated in some way and then I reassessed and started working on my next 10kgs.

So decide on what your end goal is and break it down into mini goals. It will make the task seem a lot more achievable and you won't continually stress yourself about how you're going to get to your end goal.

Think about when you hop into your car to go somewhere you haven't been before. You have a general idea, so you get in your car and drive and eventually, you get there. You may take a couple of detours or wrong turns along the way, but you do get there.

And it's the same with your weight release as long as you just keep going.

SHARI'S FAB ACTION STEP

Get out your FAB planner and write down your end goal. Then break that end goal down into smaller increments. So for instance, if you are currently a size 20 and your end goal is to be a size 14, then your mini goals could be 1 dress size. So mini goal 1 would be size 18; mini goal 2 would be size 16; and your final goal would by size 14.

KEY 8: Find What Works For YOU

If you're holding onto weight, then what you're doing is not working. If it's not working, you have to try another way. You may need to try many different things before you find what works for YOU.

When it comes to weight release there is no such thing as "one size fits all". Everyone is different. We have different body types which react in different ways to different foods. We have different likes and dislikes. We have different family units. We have different lifestyles. We have different daily responsibilities and routines. We have different budgets.

It's no wonder there are so many different weight release methods out there and unfortunately not everything works for everybody. What worked for your best friend is not necessarily going to work for you and vice versa. You might not find what works for you straight away. It might take trying a few different things to find the best fit for you and your unique set of circumstances, but it will definitely be worth it in the end.

It's a bit like buying a car. Usually we do some research and narrow the list down, then we go and have a look at the ones we've shortlisted. We sit in them. We take them for a test drive and only when we're sure it's the right car for what we need, do we make a final decision.

Finding a system of releasing weight that works for you is exactly the same. It takes time and patience, but it's totally worth the final result. So always keep in mind you may need to adapt to suit your own self and circumstances and that some methods just may not work for you at all, and that's OK!

I have tried many different things over the years. For instance, I found that counting calories worked for me at the time because it meant that I knew exactly how much I was consuming each day, as opposed to another eating plan that I tried where portion sizes weren't measured and it was very easy for me to overeat. One of my friends didn't succeed with counting calories because they felt it was too difficult for them, yet she had success with the same eating plan that I hadn't had success with.

SHARI'S FAB ACTION STEP

Get out your FAB planner and write down any eating plans or exercise regimes that have either worked for you in the past or not worked for you. Then analyse each one and try to identify why they did or didn't. This will help you when you're creating your action plan for each change that you make on your weight release journey.

KEY 9: Rome Wasn't Built in A Day – It WILL Take Time!

We get so frustrated when our weight release is slow don't we? It's frustrating to be doing all the right things and although we see progress, it just seems to take forever. When you think about it, it's ironic really. I mean, how long did it take to put the weight on in the first place? I bet it wasn't a five minute process!

As difficult as it is, try to be patient with the process. It didn't take 5 minutes to gain the weight and it won't take 5 minutes to release it, but as long as you stick at it, release it you will.

"Rome wasn't built in a day" and "slow and steady wins the race" are definitely relevant to the weight release process!

Towards the end of my weight release journey my weight release was REALLY slow! I didn't give up though. I just kept going and I got there in the end. You will too, as long as you keep going.

SHARI'S FAB ACTION STEP

Get out your FAB planner and write down some affirmations that will help you when you get frustrated along the way. Write down why you are doing this in the first place. Write down some other instances of goals you have achieved that might have taken a while but you got there in the end. Write down anything that you feel might help you when you're feeling like it's a long hard slog!

KEY 10: Don't Give Up!

Have you tried many times to release weight and not succeeded? Think about *why*. Was it because it seemed like you were never going to get to the end of your journey? Did it all seem too hard? Did you simply give up after a while?

One thing I can promise you is that as long as you keep going, you WILL get there in the end. My 100kg weight release journey was certainly not perfect and your journey won't be either. You may fall off the wagon from time to time. You may go 1 step forward and 2 steps back and trip and fall every now and then, but as long as you get back up, dust yourself off and keep going, you will always get there in the end.

Just DON'T EVER GIVE UP! The ONLY time we fail is when we give up. Otherwise there is no failure, only learning! Just take it one step at a time and one day you'll look behind you at all the steps you've taken and realise just how far you've come. Have you dusted off those pants yet?

SHARI'S FAB ACTION STEP

Get out your FAB planner and write down any inspiring success stories that you know. It doesn't have to be to do with weight release. It can be anything that you identify as being motivating and inspiring, and when you think about them, it reminds you that anything is possible. When you have those days where you feel like giving up, you can look at the examples that you've written and remind yourself that you CAN do it! Also write a list of people that you can call on for support on days where you feel as if it is all a bit too hard.

KEY 11: Lifelong Changes

The mistake that so many of us make when we try to release weight is we decide we're going on a diet or a 12-week challenge or maybe we try the latest pill or shake fad. But how long are you planning on sticking to that strict diet that you've set for yourself? How long are you going to take the pills or drink the shakes?

Everyone wants a quick fix, but none of these options are designed to be taken forever and depending on what road you've chosen, it may also not be a healthy option either. Challenges are great to get you started or remotivated along the way, but the most important thing to realise is that whatever changes you make need to be for *life*.

If you don't, what will happen is this:

You will continue the diet or the pills or the shakes until you lose weight. Then you'll go back to your normal eating, as a lot of people do. Before long, you're right back where you started. You'll have regained the weight that you lost and more. Trust me I know, because I've been there!

Always remember that this is YOUR journey and it's about finding what works for YOU in the long term. If you want to release the weight and keep it off for life, you need to identify what changes need to be made and go about implementing them one at a time in a way you can *sustain*.

You want to donate those kilos to the universe forever and not have them find you ever again! It may take you a lot longer to release the weight initially, but I promise it will be worth it in the end.

SHARI'S FAB ACTION STEP

Get out your FAB planner and write down some changes you know you need to make. Then write down beside them how you're going to do that in a way you can sustain for life.

KEY 12: The 6 Human Needs

Do you ever wonder why you continue a bad habit even when you know it's not good for you? Did you know that we have 6 human needs? They are:

- Certainty

- Variety

- Significance

- Connection

- Growth

- Contribution

For any behaviour or habit you continue on a regular basis, whether it's positive or negative, you'll find that at least 3 of the 6 human needs are being met in some way. For instance, I hate exercise. It's hard work. I get hot and sweaty. I get a red face and look extremely unattractive. Yet I exercise on average 6 days per week most weeks.

Why? Let's analyse it.

Firstly, I gain certainty from it. I am absolutely CERTAIN that it's going to help me control my weight. Secondly, I get variety from it. I go to group sessions and each session has a different trainer and each trainer trains differently. Thirdly, I get significance. I push myself to keep up with or do better than others in the session. It makes me feel good when I can see how much better my fitness level is now compared to someone who is just starting out on their fitness journey.

It also gives me connection. I connect with my trainers and my training buddies. Human need 5 – growth – I see regular growth in my training. And finally, contribution. I help to encourage and support others and especially those who are new. I remind them they have to start somewhere and that they'll get better. When they're struggling to keep going on an exercise I tell them they can do it, even if they think they can't.

In this instance, all 6 human needs are met, but for the behaviour to continue regularly, it would only have to meet 3 of them.

SHARI'S FAB ACTION STEP

Get out your FAB planner and write down any negative behaviours or habits you find yourself engaging in regularly. Maybe it's comfort eating. Maybe it's having a glass of wine or two every night with dinner. If it's something you know has become a bad habit for you and you want to stop doing it, write down what needs it's meeting. Then write down a positive behaviour or habit that meets the same needs and substitute it for the one you want to stop.

KEY 13: Why Do We Overeat?

Back in cave people days, if food was plentiful and a cave person put on a bit of fat, the fat cells would produce Leptin. Leptin is a hormone which helps to regulate appetite by signaling the brain that it's full and that it's time for the body to move. Our ancestors didn't have a problem controlling their weight because of this natural process of the body.

Unfortunately, this is not the case for a lot of people in modern times, and there's a scientific reason for it. In some people, while they may have plenty of Leptin circulating in their body, the natural effect of it is being blocked, impeding the signal to their brain that they're full. So they keep eating and eating and eating.

I can hear you asking, "What blocks the effect of Leptin?" Here comes the interesting part.

There is another hormone that's produced naturally in the body that you're probably familiar with, and that's Insulin. Increased levels of Insulin in the body can block the natural process of Leptin and cause people to overeat. Now comes the REALLY interesting part.

What causes increased levels of Insulin in the body? Eating too much sugar and flour! We all know that too much sugar and flour is bad for us, and this is why. An added problem is that the more sugar and flour you eat, the more you want. They are very addictive! Too much sugar and flour in our diet can increase our Insulin levels to the point where it reduces the ability of Leptin to control our appetite, causing us to eat more than we should. I'm not suggesting you never have any. Where's the fun in that? However, foods containing flour and sugar should definitely be "sometimes" foods, for very good reason!

SHARI'S FAB ACTION STEP

Get out your FAB planner and write down all the things you can think of that you consume on a regular basis that contain flour or sugar. This may identify some more changes you need to make that you can add to your list.

KEY 14: Low Fat is Not Better

So many of us trying to release weight try to go the "low fat" route. It sounds logical doesn't it? If we eat less fat, then we won't be as fat! Well, if we eat raspberries, are we going to turn red? Of course not! It doesn't work that way and it doesn't work that way when it comes to fat either.

We buy low fat this and low fat that. I know – I've been guilty of it in the past. Unfortunately, just because something says that it's low fat doesn't mean it's *better*. When they take the fat out of things it doesn't taste as good, so they add all kinds of sugars and chemical flavourings to make it taste better.

Sugar is the thing we should be reducing, but I will save that for later! Good healthy fats are actually an essential part of our nutritional requirements, so don't feel guilty about eating them. It's all about the type and quantity of the fat that you eat that's important.

Some of the healthy fats I eat on a regular basis are coconut oil, olive oil, avocado, salmon, fish oil, almonds and butter. I also feel more satiated by eating a higher fat diet than when I tried to cut out as much fat as possible. I definitely don't get hungry as often which is awesome!

SHARI'S FAB ACTION STEP

Get out your FAB planner and write down some healthy fats you can incorporate into your eating regime.

KEY 15: Carbs Turn to Sugar

I'm pretty sure you know that too much sugar in your diet is not good for you for a whole host of reasons. What you might not realise is eating too much of foods such as bread, rice, cereals and pasta is also not good for us and that's because it turns to sugar in the body.

You eat it, it turns to sugar which is used for energy and then if it's not all used up, what do you think happens to it? It gets converted to fat and stored somewhere on your body. If you have a weight issue, one of the first things you should do is analyse how much bread, rice, cereals and pasta you're eating, as well as sugar.

A lot of us were raised to have cereal or toast for breakfast, a sandwich for lunch and then rice, pasta or potatoes for dinner. If this is your eating regime and you're overweight, reducing these things will make a big difference.

I definitely ate WAY too much of bread, pasta and rice. I love them so much! As soon as I started to reduce how much of them I ate, I saw a massive difference in my results.

SHARI'S FAB ACTION STEP

Get out your FAB planner and write down how often you consume foods such as rice, pasta or bread. If you're eating those foods on a daily basis, analyse whether you could reduce how often you're eating them.

KEY 16: Every Day I'm Guzzlin'!

Water is vitally important. One of the simplest things you can do to aid your weight release efforts is to drink plenty of water. When you feel thirsty, you're already dehydrated, your metabolism has already slowed down and you definitely don't want that.

You want your metabolism kicking over as fast as it can, so make sure you help it out by drinking water regularly over the course of the day. If you find it hard to remember to drink water, there are a few things you can do to help you remember such as putting an alarm on your phone to go off every hour. Or you can download an app for your phone that will remind you at regular intervals to drink water.

I take my water quota with me for the day and I know that by the end of the day I have to drink all of the water I have, which means I always know if I've had enough or not. At least 8 glasses per day is the recommended amount, but the bigger you are the more you need to drink to assist your weight release. To find out how much water you should be drinking, take your weight in kg and divide it by 0.024. The resultant number is how many millilitres of water you should be drinking every day. You also need to increase your water intake by 350ml for every 30 minutes of exercise.

SHARI'S FAB ACTION STEP

Get out your FAB planner and write down how much water you need to drink each day and how you're going to remind yourself to do it if it's an issue for you.

KEY 17: Non-Food Rewards

How do you reward yourself? So often we reward ourselves with food:

"I smashed my workout today so I'm going to have a double choc muffin. I earned it!"

"I ate really well today, so I'm having ice cream for dessert."

Sound familiar? I know... I've done it too. These days I've come far enough in my journey that I don't use food as a reward anymore. Don't get me wrong, that doesn't mean that everything I put in my mouth is best for me nutritionally. I definitely do eat things that are not in my normal healthy eating regime from time to time. But I don't eat it as a reward for exercising or sticking to my nutrition plan or finishing a project or whatever else I come up with as an excuse.

It's another one of those sneaky little self sabotaging behaviours and I've learned to control it. How do you do that? Think of some non-food rewards you can indulge in when you want to reward yourself. Especially when you get to a goal. Non-food rewards can be whatever you desire, but some suggestions are a nice hot bubble bath, a massage, a new outfit or whatever else you really enjoy.

Whenever I reached a goal on my weight release journey I would celebrate in some way. I was a single parent on a tight budget and didn't buy things for myself most of the time, but I would identify something that I really wanted, even if it wasn't expensive, and when I got to my 10kg goal I would let myself have whatever I'd decided on. Sometimes it was going to the movies, sometimes it would be a new outfit or new shoes, or even just getting my hair or nails done. It made me feel so good because not only was I getting something I wanted, but I knew that I'd worked really hard for it and appreciated it all the more.

Your non-food rewards need to be things you enjoy just as much as food otherwise you won't have a reason to make the switch. For every major goal you achieve, have a set reward that really means something to you and make sure you give yourself that reward no matter what. You earned it!

SHARI'S FAB ACTION STEP

Get out your FAB planner and write down ways you can reward yourself when you reach your first mini goal. Make sure it's something really special that you're looking forward to getting.

KEY 18: Building Muscle/Protein

Eating the right amount of protein for your body is really important when you're trying to release weight or change your body composition aka converting fat to muscle. Muscle weighs more than fat, but takes up less space on the body, so by converting fat to muscle, you may not lose *weight*, but you will lose body mass and that is what we are really aiming for – to be smaller, fitter and healthier. Whilst most people want to "lose weight" what we really want to do is lose *fat*, not *weight*.

Protein plays an important role in helping us to build and retain muscle, so having protein after exercise has benefits. Additionally, having protein with every meal helps to keep you fuller for longer, especially when you combine it with a good amount of healthy fat.

Some good sources of protein are chicken, beef, fish and eggs, just to name a few and I incorporate these into my daily eating regime. I usually have eggs for breakfast, chicken with a salad for lunch and either beef or fish with vegetables for dinner. There are many other sources of protein, so decide which ones you like and try to incorporate some into every meal.

SHARI'S FAB ACTION STEP

Get out your FAB planner and write down what kinds of protein you eat on a daily basis and when. Analyse whether you feel you're eating enough and how you're going to add it in if you feel that you aren't.

KEY 19: Treats Are Acceptable

One of the biggest mindset switches you need to make when you're on your weight release journey is to understand that *you are not* on a "diet". Going on a diet implies that it's temporary. If you go on a "diet" and then go back to your former eating regime, you're going to regain the weight over a period of time.

You need to change your lifestyle. You need to make changes that you can sustain for the rest of your life, so you don't have to worry about the weight ever finding you again.

However, is it realistic to not ever put anything in your mouth ever again that might not be the healthiest nutrition wise? Of course not! The minute you tell yourself that you can't have something, what do you want more than ever?! So don't tell yourself you can't have something. Tell yourself you're choosing not to have it TODAY. Then plan when you ARE going to have it.

If you allow yourself to have treats from time to time, you'll find it a lot easier to stick to your healthy eating regime. You CAN have your cake and eat it too, as long as it's only sometimes, not all the time. In fact, you need to, or you won't last the distance.

I love rice and pasta, but they're no longer a part of my daily healthy eating regime. Most days I CHOOSE not to have it. I DO choose it have usually one day per week and I enjoy it all the more when I do because I don't have it all the time.

SHARI'S FAB ACTION STEP

Get out your FAB planner and write what treats you like to indulge in and when you're going to have them.

KEY 20: Exercise

You don't have to exercise to release weight. Many people just change their eating regime and still achieve their weight release goals. That doesn't mean you shouldn't exercise though. In fact, I would strongly encourage you to start exercising regularly, if you don't already do so.

Why? It will *speed up* your weight release. If you do a combination of cardio and weight training (body weight is fine), you'll gain muscle and lose fat which will make you smaller quicker and you'll tone your body as you release weight. Isn't that what we want?

Of course, there are *so* many benefits to exercise that I'm not even going to begin to list them here, but whether you like exercise or not, it's something you really need to find a way to work into your daily life and it will definitely help you get to your weight release goal sooner.

I don't like exercise either, but it's one of the best things I ever made myself do and I continue to do it regularly because while I don't enjoy the execution of it, I definitely enjoy the many benefits of it!

All you need to start with is 3x30 minutes per week. Try and find something you enjoy. Get the family involved or get an exercise buddy. Dancing, aqua aerobics, football, netball, walking. It doesn't matter what it is as long as you're moving!

SHARI'S FAB ACTION STEP

Get out your FAB planner and write down what kinds of exercise you could incorporate into your week and when. Start out with 3x30 minutes per week of something you feel is achievable for you.

KEY 21: It's Not All About the Scale

When we track our weight release progress, so many of us get obsessed with the number on the scale. While it can be a good motivator to see that number going down, it can seriously do our head in when it doesn't.

Unfortunately, the scale doesn't tell the whole story. There are several factors that can impact on what the scale says and not necessarily because you aren't making any progress.

For instance, if you've added in exercise to your weekly regime, you'll gain muscle which weighs more than fat. This means when you weigh in, you may either be a bit heavier, not lost at all or not lost as much as you expected. However, I can guarantee that if you were to take your measurements, you would see a positive change.

As I said previously, the terminology most people use is "weight loss", but we really want *fat* loss and there is a big difference. So don't rely on the scale as your only measure of progress if you want to give yourself the best chance of success.

Instead, take photos at regular intervals. I would suggest at either 6, 8 or 12 week intervals. Secondly, take measurements more regularly. You can do them either weekly, fortnightly or monthly, depending on your individual circumstances. Lastly, keep track of your weight, but remember it doesn't tell the whole story and that positive change is not always going to be reflected in that number you see when you step on the scales.

SHARI'S FAB ACTION STEP

Get out your FAB planner and write down how you're going to track your progress.

KEY 22: Stress

Have you ever done all the right things, eaten right and exercised, but no matter what you do you don't seem to make any progress? It's time to consider whether you're under any kind of stress.

If you're under a lot of stress, it could seriously be impacting on your weight release efforts. Whilst stress in the short term can cause a loss of appetite, long term stress can actually raise your hunger levels. When you're under chronic stress, your body will automatically go into what's known as flight or fight response, also known as "survival mode". When your body is in this mode, it will do whatever it feels it needs to survive and that can mean overeating.

Basically, your body thinks it has used calories to fight or flee and it feels as if it needs to replenish them. Add to this the fact that there's a stress hormone called cortisol, levels of which increase in the body during times of high tension, and your overeating can turn into a habit.

Increased levels of cortisol also cause increased levels of insulin which cause your blood sugar to drop and you crave sugary, fatty foods. What kinds of foods do you usually turn to when you're under stress? I bet it is not an apple or salad! Don't you usually go for comfort foods?

The shortened version of the story is this:

More stress = more cortisol = a higher appetite for comfort food = more body fat.

When the body is in fight or flight mode, it will also shut down any processes it doesn't need, such as burning fat, in case you need to run from danger or fight it. So if you're having trouble releasing weight and you're under a lot of stress, you need to find a way to alleviate some of that stress to get your weight release moving in the right direction. You can use yoga, meditation, massage or whatever else works as a stress reliever for you.

I had a lot of stress in my life. Work, financial, family stress, you name it. I found that when I made genuine efforts to deal with it by taking time out for myself to read or meditate, my weight release seemed to be much easier.

SHARI'S FAB ACTION STEP

Get out your FAB planner and write down what kinds of stress you might be under and what you can do to relieve it in some way.

KEY 23: Sleep

Sleep is so important, even more so when we're trying to release weight. Lack of sleep affects our hormones and there are three in particular I'll talk about here.

The first one is called Grehlin. Grehlin is the hormone that tells our brain we're hungry and that it's time to eat. Lack of sleep causes the body to produce more Grehlin, so we feel hungrier.

The second one is called Leptin. Leptin is the hormone that tells our brain we're full. Sleep deprivation causes Leptin levels to drop massively and so our brain doesn't get the signal that we've had enough to eat.

The effect of these two hormones is our brain keeps thinking we're hungry and we never feel full so we eat more and more and more.

Added to that, the third hormone that comes into play is called Cortisol, the stress hormone we talked about earlier. Sleep deprivation causes a spike in Cortisol which tells our body to conserve our energy to fuel our waking hours, which means we hang onto fat.

Can you see why lack of sleep can be a huge contributor for those who have a weight problem? The amount of sleep we need to get varies from person to person, between 6 and 9 hours of sleep per night, but the bare minimum is 6 hours. Any less than that and all of the above comes into play.

When I was really overweight, I got very little sleep. Some nights I only got 3 or 4 hours. When I learned that lack of sleep could hinder weight release, I did some more research, found out that the bare minimum that I should be getting was 6 hours and made a concerted effort to get no less than 6 hours sleep per night from then on. I wasn't always successful, but I was consistent enough that I saw a definite improvement in my weight release results!

If you have a weight problem and regularly get less than 6 hours of sleep per night, do yourself a favour and find a way to get more sleep. It will benefit you in so many ways! How many hours of sleep do you average per night?

SHARI'S FAB ACTION STEP

Get out your FAB planner and write down how many hours of sleep per night you get on a regular basis. If it's less than 6 hours, how could you get at least 6 hours per night?

KEY 24: Negative Self Talk

How do you talk to yourself? Not out loud necessarily, I'm talking about the internal dialogue that, if you're anything like me, goes a mile a minute at least 20 hours of the day. Is it negative or positive?

The way we speak to ourselves quite often is utterly atrocious! If you eat something you shouldn't, do you tell yourself off about how you shouldn't have done that? How you just can't stick to a plan? How you're never going to get anywhere because you just can't control what you put in your mouth? When you can't drag yourself out of bed to go to the gym, do you tell yourself that you're lazy or useless?

I've been guilty of it, too. Let me ask you this - would you say those things to another person? If you heard someone speaking to your best friend like that, what would you do? Would you tell them not to speak to people that way? We shouldn't speak to ourselves that way either. We need to pull ourselves up when we start to become negative and immediately flip it into a positive.

One way we can do that is to replace the word "should" with "could". When you say you "should" have done this, or you "should" have done that, you're making yourself wrong for *not* doing it, and that's a negative state to be in. However, if you "could" have done it, then you're not wrong and that's a much more positive state.

You also still "could" do better next time. So what "could" you do to remind yourself to speak kindly to yourself?

Also, you'll notice throughout this book I use the term "release weight", rather than "lose weight". Did you wonder why? It's because when we lose something, what do we usually try to do? We usually try to find it again. Whereas, if we release something, we're letting it go voluntarily and happily and we don't want to go looking for it again. It's gone.

Can you see how your language could be helping or hindering you?

SHARI'S FAB ACTION STEP

Get out your FAB planner and write down any negative self talk you know goes on in your head on a regular basis. How can you turn it around and make it positive self talk instead?

KEY 25: Overeating is About Self Hate, Not Self Love

Quite often when we have a weight issue it's because we don't love ourselves. Overeating is not about gluttony or selfishness. Rather it's a way of sabotaging ourselves because we have limiting beliefs such as we're not important, we're not worthy, we're not enough or we're not loved.

Many of us don't even realise we have these limiting beliefs. When we love ourselves, it's easier to make the changes we need to make to become healthier and the weight will start to come off.

Louise Hay had a morning ritual where she would go to the mirror as soon as she got out of bed, look at herself and tell her reflection how much she loved herself. Start telling yourself how much you love yourself. You ARE important, you ARE enough, you ARE worthy and you ARE loved!

I do this every single day and every single day I love myself more and more!

SHARI'S FAB ACTION STEP

Get out your FAB planner and write down how you're going to show yourself self love on a daily basis.

KEY 26: You Are Important

So many of us spend so much time doing things for others; our children, our partner, our friends and extended family. Sometimes we spend so much time doing for others, that we don't do things for ourselves. I have on many occasions had mothers tell me they feel guilty for taking time out to spend time on their health and fitness because they feel as if it's time they should be spending doing things for their family.

My argument to that is this...

I have no doubt that most parents want to be the absolute best parent they can be for their children. One of the biggest things I came to understand was it was important for me to take the time out to do the things I needed to do to release the weight in order to be the best parent I could be. So I could run around and do things with my children. So I could teach them by example how to eat healthy and the importance of being active. I missed out on so much with my children in the years I was morbidly obese and I can never get those years back.

Realise that *you* are important, too. It's so important that you take the time out to do the things you need to do in relation to your health so you can be the best person you can be for yourself and your family.

SHARI'S FAB ACTION STEP

Get out your FAB planner and write down all the reasons why it's important for you to make the changes to become the healthiest you for you and your loved ones.

KEY 27: Planning

You've heard the saying, "Fail to plan and you plan to fail" right? Well when it comes to weight release, that saying is particularly relevant. The biggest favour you can do for yourself when you're trying to release weight is to plan and prepare your food ahead of time.

It actually makes things a whole lot easier and quicker and it can save you money. Who doesn't want more time and money?! The best thing I ever did was start planning and prepping food ahead of time. Each week I sit down with my daughter before shopping day and we plan the food we're eating for the next week. Then we make the shopping list based on what we need for our meals that week and I go and do the shopping. Then we batch cook to save time.

It makes it cheaper because we only buy what we need for that week and it saves time because we make enough food for a few days at a time, so we only have to cook a few times a week.

When you have a busy life, as so many of us do, it can make life so much easier. It also makes it easier to stay on track with your food because you already have a healthy meal prepared that you can grab whenever you need.

SHARI'S FAB ACTION STEP

Get out your FAB planner and write down what you're going to plan and how. Will it be your food? Will it be your exercise?

KEY 28: Accountability

If you really want to achieve your weight release goals, accountability is an important factor and can take many different forms. It could be in the form of logging everything you put in your mouth to make you accountable to yourself. You could take it one step further and ask someone to be your accountability partner and show it to them once a week.

If you know you're going to have to show it to someone each week, you'll think twice before you eat something you shouldn't or skip your planned exercise routine. Weight Watchers or some other kind of weight release support group where you regularly have an official weigh in can also be great for accountability and you could do the same with an accountability partner. You could also have your accountability partner take your measurements once a month. Another option is to hire a personal trainer or a weight release coach or mentor to be accountable to.

If you know you'll struggle at times to stay on track, think about some form of accountability that will help you to keep on the straight and narrow.

SHARI'S FAB ACTION STEP

Get out your FAB planner and write down how you are going to stay accountable.

KEY 29: Support

The task of releasing weight is at times not an easy one. There are lots of things that can help along the way and one of the biggest ones is having support. In particular, support in the form of a buddy or weight release partner can be really helpful. A mentor can also be a massive form of support. It can be someone that you know who has successfully navigated the same journey you are on, or a paid coach or mentor.

Your buddy can either be on their own weight release mission, or you can simply have a caring friend or family member as a buddy. Either way, that person should be someone you can talk to about the highs and lows, someone that will help keep you on track and accountable, someone that will make you keep your promise to get out of bed and exercise if that's in your plan.

Your buddy is your biggest cheerleader. They have the tough job of helping to keep you positive when the road gets tough. They will help you up when you fall down and give you a massive hug when you need it. The support that you receive from your family and friends is what helps you to keep going, especially on those really tough days. They can't do the work for you, but they can encourage you and remind you of how amazing you are during those times when you forget how amazing you are.

You aren't on your own, although you will sometimes feel as if you are and that's when having encouraging and supportive people around you will help you immensely. Every time someone notices you've made progress and comments on it, every time someone tells you they're proud of you and to keep going, every time someone doesn't recognise you because they haven't seen you for a while, every time someone tells you that you're looking utterly FABulous, the smile gets a little bit wider... the step gets a little lighter... and the self belief grows that little bit more.

I had a lot of support on my journey and I am so grateful for all of it. I also had a beautiful lady mentoring me at my local curves, I learned so much from her and she gave me so much encouragement and support. Of course all the ladies that worked there were extremely encouraging and supportive, but this one in particular went the extra mile.

I remember one particular weigh and measure with her was when I was trying to get to double digits on the scale. I was so close and I knew there was a slight difference in the scales at Curves and my scales at home. I got on my scales at home and I had double digits, but only just and I knew that I weighed a couple of hundred grams more on the Curves scales.

I was so excited! I raced to Curves, ran in, ran down to the back of the room and picked up the scales and went to find Soozie. I had an excited grin on my face and she looked at me wondering what was going on because I had the scales in my hand. I said "Soozie, I have a massive favour to ask!" She asked me what it was. I asked if we could do my weigh in in the change room, so she could look down at the scales and close her eyes and just open them when I told her to without looking up. She laughed! She realized that I might need to take my clothes off! She said for me, she would do it, because she knew what goal I was trying to get to. We went into the change room, she got into position and closed her eyes. I hopped on clothed and was 200g over. I knew I would be! So I told her I was taking some clothes off. I ended up having to take all of them off, was stark naked, saw the double digits on the scale, told her to open her eyes, she saw and then closed her eyes again while I redressed. When I was suitably attired, she opened her eyes and we jumped up and down together, laughing and crying. She was so happy for me. That kind of support is INVALUABLE!

So get that cheer squad sorted, because they're an important part of the process!

SHARI'S FAB ACTION STEP

Get out your FAB planner and write down who you could ask to be a part of your cheer squad!

KEY 30: A Total Mind, Body, Spirit Approach

Successful long term weight release takes a total mind, body, spirit approach. It's not all about nutrition and exercise. It takes a combination of working on your mindset, your nutrition, physical movement and self love and care. Different people will find different tools to help them not only release the weight, but to keep it off long term. You never know what tool or modality is going to help you in some way, so keep an open mind and be prepared to try different things. If it doesn't work, let it go, but if it helps in some way, then add it into your routine.

Over the years I have added in things such as meditation and network spinal analysis. I have created a "success ritual" for myself that I carry out daily which includes self love practices, envisioning and affirmations. These things help to keep me focused on my goals every single day.

SHARI'S FAB ACTION STEP

Get out your FAB planner and write down the different things you haven't tried that you feel could be helpful on your weight release journey, such as meditation, yoga, massage, etc.

KEY 31: Education

Education is so important when it comes to our health and wellness. There is new research all the time and it's hard to keep up with it. For instance, for many years all the experts taught that low fat was the best way to go, whilst in recent times studies have shown that it's really certain carbohydrates we need to reduce and we actually need good quality healthy fats in our diet.

It can be very confusing at times, but as long as you're open to learning and trying new things, then you'll have a much better chance of finding what works for you. Remember, a parachute works best when it's open.

I've learned so much on my own weight release journey and I continue to learn every day. When I learn something new, I give it a try and if it works for me I keep it and if it doesn't, I don't. So much of what I am teaching in this book and to my clients is stuff that I learned along my own journey that I tried, found worked and kept and I know that this process will keep repeating for the rest of my life.

SHARI'S FAB ACTION STEP

Get out your FAB planner and write down some ways that you could learn more about health and wellness.

One Change at A Time

I know there probably seems like a whole lot you need to change to reach your weight release goal, but please don't forget the number one rule with all of this. ONE CHANGE AT A TIME!

Yes, I did really just yell at you! It came from a place of love and understanding though. Please know that you have absolutely everything inside of you to change your story one change at a time.

Yes, it will take time. Yes, there will be detours. Sometimes you may feel like you're taking one step forward and two back. Know that as long as you don't give up, as long as you keep going, you will absolutely get to your destination in the end.

Whatever that destination is for you, it will be perfect just for you. It will be amazing and wonderful and everything that you thought it would be and oh so much more. That's how it was for me and that's what I know is possible for you, as long as you believe.

Belief in yourself is such a powerful thing. You can do anything you put your mind to if you want it enough and believe in yourself enough. Anything is possible. I have proven that and so many others in the world have as well. We are not more unique than you. We are no more special than you. We are human beings just like you who made a decision to change and stuck with it because we wanted it so much and believed we could do it.

Now it's your turn. So what are you waiting for? Go forth and conquer and all that good stuff. Find your WHY! Identify your why nots. BELIEVE you CAN change your story one change at a time! Set your goal, identify the changes you need to make and get started on the first one.

It's time. It's time for *you*. It's time for you to make yourself a priority. It's time for you to do things for yourself that will make your life better, which will in turn improve the lives of all of those around you. It's time for you to show yourself what you're made of. You are strong. You are unbeatable. You are bloody AMAZING!

I truly hope that my story has been of help to you. I know where you're at. I know how you got there. I know where you want to go and I know you can get there. No one can do it for you. The only person who can change YOUR story is YOU... and change it you will!

Always remember, the only time we fail is when we give up. So don't give up on YOU! There is a beautiful life full of joy and happiness and health and fun out there waiting for you. So get in your car, start the engine and get moving in the right direction. Have fun along the way. You will laugh. You will cry. You will hurt. You will make yourself so damn proud!

You know you can do it. Yes YOU! The world is waiting for you! It's time for YOU to find YOUR FABulous!

To help you carry on with your journey, there are two options for your next step. Firstly you can connect with me on any of my social media here:

Connect with me on Facebook:

https://www.facebook.com/shariwarefab

Connect with me on my Facebook Page:

https://www.facebook.com/fabnewbody

Connect with me on Instagram:

https://www.instagram.com/shariwarefab

Connect with me on Twitter: https://twitter.com/shariwarefab

Connect with me on Linked In:

https://www.linkedin.com/in/shariware

And if you're ready to find YOUR FABulous today, contact me for a complimentary 30 minute chat to get you started:

You can book in here: https://calendly.com/shari-ware/30min

The support of a mentor, especially at the beginning of your journey, is invaluable and I was so lucky to have the beautiful Soozie mentoring me and supporting me on mine. I can't even put into words how grateful I am for the understanding, advice, support and encouragement that she gave me. So take the first step towards FABulous today!

About the Author

SHARI WARE

PERSONAL LIFESTYLE RENOVATION SPECIALIST

Personal Lifestyle Renovation Specialist and #1 Best Selling Author Shari Ware went from slicing a piece of cake, to slicing her weight in half! In fact, she spent more than a decade in the morbidly obese classification and was fortunate that no major health crisis came her way.

Shari now helps others win the weight battle the way she did – one change at a time. Shari has made it her mission to help others change their story and find their HEALTHY. She discovered the secret to successfully releasing weight and found that it applies to every goal that we set for ourselves in life. Now she helps others to find their WHY Power as a critical starting point which, in conjunction with making a series of changes over a period of time, leads to massive change.

Other tools that Shari has added to her toolbelt to help people are a Personal Training qualification and a certification in Hypnotherapy, NLP and Life Coaching. She's been featured by That's Life Magazine, Take 5 and New Idea as well as appearing on Today Tonight, the Channel 9 Morning Show and Channel 9 News.

Shari has also been featured in various Australian and UK online news publications such as The Telegraph and The Courier Mail.

If you would like to connect with Shari and find out how she helps people to overcome Mephobia and change their story in various ways, including helpful and practical tips, you can do so on Facebook at:

https://www.facebook.com/fabnewbody

I hope you enjoyed this book! Please feel free to share it with friends and post a review so I can help more people to find THEIR healthy!

Shari Ware

Personal Lifestyle Renovation Specialist

xoxo

DON'T FORGET TO:

Book a complimentary 30-minute call with me to find your healthy!

https://calendly.com/shari-ware/30min

Connect with me on Facebook – Shari Ware

https://www.facebook.com/shariwarefab

Connect with me on Facebook – FAB New Body

https://www.facebook.com/fabnewbody

Connect with me on Instagram

https://www.instagram.com/shariwarefab

Connect with me on Twitter

https://twitter.com/shariwarefab

Connect with me on Linked In

https://www.linkedin.com/in/shariware

#1 Best Selling Author of Healthy! Beautiful Inside & Out

You can get the book here: https://amzn.to/2V1LXfg